Statistical Methods in Neuropsychology

David Aaron Maroof

Statistical Methods in Neuropsychology

Common Procedures Made Comprehensible

Springer

David Aaron Maroof
The Esplanade 8767
Orlando, FL, USA

ISBN 978-1-4614-3416-0 e-ISBN 978-1-4614-3417-7
DOI 10.1007/978-1-4614-3417-7
Springer New York Heidelberg Dordrecht London

Library of Congress Control Number: 2012934669

Printed on acid-free paper

Springer is part of Springer Science+Business Media (www.springer.com)

Preface

I realize that given the miscegenation between neuropsychology and statistics, dovetailing the two into a book, this book, would be a step in the right direction. That step includes the explaining of several of the uses and purposes of some very common statistical analyses. My intention is to simplify material that is all too often, perhaps unwittingly, bemused by authors who place greater emphasis on the mathematical algorithms and principles that underpin statistical analyses rather than simply describing their applications, limitations, and interpretations. My own discontent, as well as that of my colleagues' and students', with such common enterprises of concealing statistical knowledge in a mass of technical hugger-mugger—disaffects most—but it has only waxed my interest. The result is this Book.

This is not the first and only foray into providing a more practical and concrete explication of common statistical strategies. However, this book remains distinctive in that it provides unsophisticated explanations of statistics with examples of neuropsychological inquiries. I am hopeful that this book will provide the reader with a basic, yet fundamental understanding of these methods; and that this knowledge will serve as a springboard with which he can accomplish more challenging statistics

Orlando, FL, USA David Aaron Maroof

Acknowledgments

I would like to for express my gratitude to those who gave me the imprimatur and encouraged me to embark on this journey.

My wife, Anju, was tremendous in bringing me to heel whenever I exhibited an occasional temper tantrum while writing this book (it happens to the best of us). And, our children, Jacob and Rayna: there is nothing more humbling and impressive than spending time with you. May your lives continue to upstage mine in every way, shape and form. I love you.

I would also like to thank all my professors from Yeshiva University, my supervisors while on internship at Jersey Shore University Medical Center, in particular Dr. Angelica Diaz-Martinez, as well as faculty throughout my fellowship in clinical neuropsychology at Johns Hopkins University School of Medicine. In some way, you have all helped to transform an inchoate interest into an indelible passion. And for that, I thank you all.

Contents

Chapter 1
Introduction

Relinquishing the Sturm and Drang of Learning Statistics

So you have chosen to read a book about the application of statistical tests to clinical neuropsychological research. To reward you for such a wise, yet inexorably painful journey, I have decided to explain the material herein with minimal use of mathematical precepts or statistical jargon. After having taught several courses (both undergraduate and graduate), I have come to realize that the best ways of approaching such dense and obscure material—or any material for that matter—are with plain English and simple examples. Statistics is all too often presented, in byzantine abstractions and inkhorn language. However, descriptions should clarify, not mystify.

That neuropsychology compels one to develop a firm understanding of primer level and perhaps more advanced statistical wherewithal is certain. Students and clinicians often hang on tenterhooks when faced with statistics, whether it is to read or apply such methods. For students, it is often in class or when faced with analyses of a dissertation; for clinicians, it is when reading or conducting research to stay abreast of current practice or to grapple with a thorny clinical case.

Simply passing a statistics course by a hair's breadth in graduate school will not suffice when one is out in the real world. Why would it? Passing a statistics course with an excellent grade is equally disadvantageous when it is based merely on plugging numbers into formulae that generate, by way of a process akin to thaumaturgy, statistics that putatively symbolize clinically relevant information. Unfortunately, this is usually par for the course. An excellent mark will look nice on your transcript, but will serve no other purpose.

Understanding statistical methods most often used in neuropsychological research and practice will place one in a much better position of being capable of impugning, demystifying, or debunking a neuropsychological theory, the reason being that the majority of clinical practice is tethered to empirical studies: these studies rely on statistical design and analysis to confirm or disconfirm theories between brain–behavior relationships.

D.A. Maroof, *Statistical Methods in Neuropsychology: Common Procedures Made Comprehensible*, DOI 10.1007/978-1-4614-3417-7_1,

Those who find delving into the realm of statistics too daunting will be hamstrung in his efforts to fully appreciate clinical neuropsychology. It is foolish to remain in class, or in clinical practice, in such high dudgeon when faced with statistics. This type of professional stonewalling is useless. It is in your best interest to gain a better appreciation of statistics: what they are, what they mean, and why they are used.

As I mentioned most courses in statistics are taught with an emphasis on the clandestine mathematics of statistical procedures, including convoluted matrix algebra. Unless you plan on earning a doctorate in mathematics, I see no purpose in reviewing—or reliving—the mathematical principles driving these statistical models. And, I am not attempting to present myself as a self-styled statistician. What matters in the "real world" (and the real world for me is in the clinical neuropsychology world) is not being able to reel off mathematical algorithms. Rather, an understanding of statistics at a basic conceptual and practical level is likely more constructive for our purposes.

There is also no need to hide behind highfalutin or turgid language to explain the principal concepts in most statistical analyses. Bombastic prose serves its purpose, but not when trying to comprehend material that is inherently abstract.

Now we have user-friendly software packages that allow for extremely brisk and efficient data analysis. Software packages can handle a tremendous amount of throughput in a matter of seconds, and the results are displayed so rapidly that we (maybe just me) experience some semblance of compunction at their simplicity. The value of software packages—and point and click methods of data analysis—is that they allow us to reallocate our focus back onto more worthwhile endeavors: understanding the conceptual underpinnings of statistical techniques.

While I was in graduate school, my professors would lament about their own experiences in graduate school ("back in the day"). They did not have the convenience of software packages, and were left with handheld calculators to tackle statistical analyses. I am sure there was some benefit to working on research in this way, but I must be too myopic to see it right now. Students and researchers have enough difficulty generating solid hypotheses and interpreting output. By having researchers continue with the use of handheld calculators would only add insult to injury and would likely detract from time better spent understanding why we do what we do.

I also hope to infuse some of this book with a bit of humor. I find that using jokes often dampens the gravity and torture of a topic, especially a topic that is all too often considered anathema to most people because of its seeming complexity; this reputation has made statistics the bête noire of students and clinicians.

Other than humor, there are other ways to help learn material. Once I have your guard down with my winning personality, I will hit you with an additional trick up my sleeve: concrete examples. I am hopeful that my overly simplistic examples will at least convey that learning such material need not be as agonizing as previously thought. In school, we learn so much about the real world without gaining the exposure. I guess this is as presumptuous as thinking your skill in street combat would be honed if you were to watch The Karate Kid. You get the point. I will show you the real world, with simple example.

This is not to say that statistics is not a complex matter. However, we need not understand everything at a molecular level! For example, a healthy lifestyle (by eating right and exercising) makes sense at face value; most do not comprehend the complex physiology behind why and how healthy behaviors are, well, healthy. This applies to learning statistics, which does not require knowledge of its inner mechanics. However, a sense of humor is imperative.

In the end, you can boast a general knowledge for something that has always been considered foreign and impenetrable. You will be more confident and perhaps somewhat more capable when confronted with a statistical dilemma.

You need only read. This is not wrestling. There is no need to dodge convoluted mathematical formulae (there are none, your welcome), or trip over the meanings of large words such as *heteroscedasticity* (I will explain them in due time). Why make material that is by its very nature abstract, even more so? I do not need to impress you with large words (I am no sesquipedalian), or hide behind fanciful terminology. If I wanted to impress you, I would have written an autobiography! I have no desire to expatiate on every minute detail, but rather to provide an overall sense of the methods used and what they do.

Do not attempt to read this entire book holus-bolus. Read and re-read this book, or each chapter, using a piecemeal approach. Some topics may be more difficult for you to grasp than others—spend more time with those areas.

I would not expect you to complete this book with a full knowledge of statistics. I do not have a full knowledge of statistics. Rather, I expect that you become more cognizant of commonly used statistical techniques that are applied within the field of clinical neuropsychology, to understand why they have been chosen to analyze particular hypotheses (with particular data), and more importantly, what they mean.

This book is not intended as a cookbook for how to go about data analysis. No two studies are identical, and therefore, should not be treated as such. After all, there are several books already devoted to data analysis (e.g., George & Mallery, 2007; Green & Salkind, 2005).

All joking aside, I want to thank you for deciding that this book was worth your while to purchase, borrow, pilfer, whatever. I hope that I am able to dovetail neuropsychology and statistics into a manner that is coherent, concise, and perhaps palatable. Enjoy!

Chapter 2
Validity

Introduction

Before I discuss the importance of validity and how it relates to those who practice clinical neuropsychology, a definition is in order. Validity is an umbrella term with many tributaries, all of which have slightly different meanings and methods for determining their legitimacy (Nunnally & Bernstein, 1994). However, the linchpin of all validation studies in neuropsychology is the ability to operationally define and uncover unique dimensions of cognitive architecture that serve to describe, explain, and predict. Real-world experiences (including affect, behavior, and cognition) are sampled by neuropsychological tests. Thus, someone who experiences word-finding difficulties in conversation is likely to demonstrate such difficulties on tests of naming (e.g., the Boston Naming Test) (Kaplan, Goodglass, & Weintrab, 1983). This test, among all tests in neuropsychology, is predicated on the assumption that occurrences outside of the examination room are captured on neuropsychological testing, and that these measures represent bona fide surrogates for "life experiences" and brain function. This is validity.

Hypothetical Constructs

A hypothetical construct is something believed to exist despite an inability to measure or observe this phenomenon directly. As in psychodynamic thought where we are faced with unobservable, latent constructs such as the id, ego, and superego, in neuropsychology, we must reconcile with what we are unable to assess unalloyed phenomena—including anxiety and executive cognition. Despite neuropsychology's appearance of perhaps more "scientific" and quantifiable pursuits (e.g., akin to the physical sciences), we are still left in the uncanny position of having to develop measures that serve as proxies for a plethora of neuropsychological constructs such as memory, attention, as well as spatial, configural, and executive cognition.

D.A. Maroof, *Statistical Methods in Neuropsychology: Common Procedures Made Comprehensible*, DOI 10.1007/978-1-4614-3417-7_2,

Since neuropsychologists are compelled into indirect observation, they must backpedal and determine whether the methods cultivated to quantify and measure neuropsychological constructs are indeed measuring what they are claimed to measure.

Fundamentally, neuropsychologists want to ensure that the constructs measured are the sole cause of variability in test performance: depression (or lack thereof) causes scores on a scale for depression to fluctuate, as an example. And, if someone is having problems with attention, then this difficulty presumably should be exerting a causal influence on tests requiring attention and concentration. Thus, test are themselves the operational definitions for the constructed they measure.

But, What Is Validity?

As in any other discipline, the overarching definition of validity within neuropsychology has to do with authenticity—do our tests, scales, indices, measures, etc. measure what we say they measure? Does a list learning test measure memory? Does an index that we have developed to measure depression, actually measure depression, and if so, does it measure different aspects of depression, such as affect (feelings of sadness), behavior (social withdrawal), and cognition (negative thoughts)?

Even if we have established that our measures adequately embody these hypothetical constructs, assessing what we want them to, can they reliably distinguish among disorders? These are important empirical questions that we must try to answer in order to ensure neuropsychology as a worthy science. These are questions that can be addressed with validation studies.

This book (or chapter) does not cover reliability, which is the consistency in one's measurement. However, validity presupposes reliability. On the other hand, a measure can be reliable and yet still entirely invalid. For example, suppose I were to say that hopping on one foot is a reliable measure of intelligence. This may be reliable (if someone can hop on his or her foot for 1 min, they will be or likely to be able to do the same task sometime in the near future). However, it is very unlikely that hopping on one foot is a valid measure of intelligence (in fact, if someone hops on one foot thinking that it is measuring intelligence, then, I guess we are measuring something else (e.g., gullibility?)).

What Are the Types of Validity?

There are several aspects of validity, including content, criterion, construct, incremental, and ecological validity. Validity is a process. It is equally important to remember that validity is a function of the context in which a test is used; it is not entirely tied or attributed to the makeup of a test. It takes two to Tango. Thus, using a test of rapid motor responding in someone with hemiplegia is inappropriate. In this case, it is not the test that is invalid, but the context, which is unsuitable.

As I mentioned, establishing the validity of neuropsychological measures is a process. Items to be included in an instrument considered to reflect the hypothetical construct must be selected (content validity). This can be conceived somewhat as a form of face validity—do the questions or items we have devised seem to measure what we want to measure? However, content validity generally requires more scientific verification. Following decisions on the items for inclusion, the next step may be to determine whether these items truly measure what they are supposed to be measuring (construct validity). This involves examining two important lines of evidence. First, is our construct associated with other measures that assess the same construct (convergent validity)? Second, is our construct unrelated to other measures that should have no relation to our construct (divergent validity)? This can be a somewhat difficult endeavor in neuropsychology because, as you are well aware, many measures in neuropsychology are correlated with one another. Another crucial step in the validation process is to ascertain whether test scores predict conceptually related outcomes. For example, does a scale that measures impulsivity and poor decision making correctly classify those who are incarcerated or involved in other illegal activity?

Two other important method, incremental and ecological validity, minister to clinical neuropsychology. Incremental validity examines how well the addition of certain tests aids in explaining the variation in the dependent variable. For example, does including motivation in an analysis have significant weight in predicting academic achievement over and above intelligence and/or traditional cognitive testing?

Ecological validity on the other hand examines whether neuropsychological tests and constructs relate to real-world functioning. Does a test of executive cognition really reflect someone's ability to reason and problem solve in everyday life (e.g., would a neuropsychological test indicate whether an individual would know what to do should his or her car breakdown?)? Tests that mimic daily functioning (e.g., writing checks or finding phone numbers in a simulated phonebook) have been developed in an effort to offer more face valid assessments with the hopes of capturing how a person actually handles such matters outside of testing. This is an important enterprise for neuropsychologists as neuropsychological testing is often solicited to speculate or render fail-safe decisions on a person's ability to function in a variety of capacities (e.g., live on his or her own versus some form of congregate housing).

Classify or Predict? What's the Big Deal?

Although often used as synonyms, the terms "classify" and "predict" should not be used interchangeably. One is not necessarily predicting something when using data (both test scores and outcome measures)—such as in a regression analysis—that were collected simultaneously. So, if patients with Alzheimer's disease and healthy persons were evaluated on a neuropsychological battery, and then it is determined which tests help discriminate the two groups, the researcher is not really predicting group membership per se. Instead, he or she is classifying or merely distinguishing between two groups. There is no temporal component to this study, and therefore, this is more of a classification procedure.

The term "predict" should be used, for instances in which the outcome/criterion (such as disease) develops subsequent to measurement of a particular phenomenon. In this sense, prediction means that a score or someone's performance on a particular measure augurs for the person's status (outcome), much like the genetic mutation for Huntington's disease predicts that a person will develop HD—though, not when the person might develop manifest HD (the onset of symptoms). However, when sufficient control is exerted over a number of factors, this bolsters the researcher's confidence that particular tests or findings portend a specific outcome. Thus, knowledge of one piece of information (e.g., test performance) foretells the advent of a particular outcome. It can then be concluded that test performance predicts an outcome with a reasonable degree of certainty.

As another example, patients with Alzheimer disease perform worse on many measures than would normal controls. However, if a cohort of elderly individuals, all healthy, were to complete a neuropsychological battery, and then were followed prospectively, the researcher could establish who develops Alzheimer disease over a certain period of time. The researcher can then determine whether any of the tests the participants completed at baseline predict their *current* status. Here, we can say that a test (or tests) score predicted disease outcome. Note that this is not the same as saying a score *caused* the outcome to occur. Rather, the scores at baseline were likely the cause of a percolating, yet unapparent, inconspicuous illness.

Now let us turn to exploring validity in a bit more detail. While there are other types of validity (e.g., internal, external) we focus on five I mentioned above: content, criterion, construct, incremental, and ecological.

Content Validity

Content validity has to do with how well an instrument is able to capture and encompass all the conceptual aspects of a construct. The researcher must ensure that the items selected for his instrument are an adequate sample from some theoretical content domain. In other words, to assess anxiety, all elements of this construct (physiological, behavioral, and affective) must be included in a measure. However, most researchers in neuropsychology find that the majority of constructs are overly broad; they recognize that to develop one scale or measure to assess every component of a construct would be equally difficult and would likely dilute the significance and meaning of that very construct. This is why more specific aspects of functioning are conceptualized (e.g., set-shifting), rather than tests that measure expansive constructs such as executive functioning proper.

Let us use an example of depression to describe the development of a scale's content validity. The question remains: Is the instrument capturing the affective, behavioral, and cognitive components of depression? There are two methods for which to judge content validity, subjective and objective.

The subjective process would involve asking "experts" within the domain of interest (e.g., depression) to review the instrument's items and decide whether it does indeed cover all aspects of this construct.

An objective measure might be the use of factor analysis to verify the domains that the measure is tapping into. So, after items for the scale have been constructed, and it has been administered to a sample, a factor analysis should reveal the three domains that the instrument was expected to encompass: affective, behavioral, and cognitive dimensions. This is content validity because the measure *fits* with the concept (and content) of depression.

Criterion Validity

Criterion validity has to do with how well an instrument predicts or is associated with an observed indicator of a given concept or criterion (Bryant, 2000). If the measure is genuinely measuring a particular construct, like memory, then, its classification and predictive ability should be well established. An instrument must have an empirical association with some conceptually related criterion.

If a newly developed measure of memory is in fact measuring memory, it should differentiate among persons with amnestic mild cognitive impairment (those with memory deficits only) and those who are cognitively intact. Similarly, if on a measure of daily living skills and independence, one's performance correlates well with his or her real-life adaptive functioning, this demonstrates criterion validity. If a person who is dependent in everyday life, but breezes through the test, then this test may lack criterion validity.

A measure can lack criterion validity for several reasons. First, the content of items (content validity) might be insufficient. Second, the items may not reflect the complexity of real life. For example, people often have much structure in performing tasks when undergoing neuropsychological assessment, whereas they often have to recall and initiate many tasks on their own in real life. One might say that this measure lacks ecological validity—how well a person's performance on neuropsychological testing mirrors or represents how he performs outside of the testing room (cf. Chaytor & Schmitter-Edgecombe, 2003). There are methods for assessing criterion validity, all of which have to do with the temporal ordering of measurement. These approaches include retrospective (postdictive), concurrent, and predictive/prospective validity.

Retrospective/Postdictive Validity

Retrospective validity is fraught with several methodological flaws. The problem with this type of validity is that a construct—a behavior for example—is measured in hindsight, after it has actually occurred. In neuropsychology, a researcher might be interested in looking at the effects of maternal alcohol abuse during pregnancy and their offspring's performance on cognitive testing at 18 years of age. Thus, tests of the teenagers' current cognitive functioning are possible, but the researcher must rely on available archival data and self-report for additional information (i.e., while their mothers were pregnant). This information might be inaccessible, as it may include acquiring information with regard to how much their mother was drinking at pregnancy, how often, during which trimester (s), and all other salient factors considered might be relevant both during the pregnancy of the mother as well as throughout the course of the participant's (offspring's) development.

Another example would be to compare patients' intellectual function as adults with the number of school absences as a child. The neuropsychologist could assess a group's intellectual function, and then obtain school records from their respective elementary, middle, and high schools. A hypothesis might be that, limiting the study to high school graduates, and controlling for age or significant life-altering factors in school (health problems or family issues), the number of absences is inversely related to adult IQ. That is, the higher the IQ, the less likely the person missed school.

Generally, correlational and regression analyses are appropriate for establishing a measure's postdictive validity. If the variables of interest are highly correlated, or one has significant predictive power, then this supports a measure's postdictive validity.

Unfortunately, there are a number of methodological flaws with postdictive validity. One problem, as you can already imagine, is that memories for past information are subject to massive gaps and distortions. In some cases, archival data (e.g., medical charts) might help reconcile some of these problems.

Concurrent Validity

In this case, the test score and the outcome variable are measured concurrently. For example, one can examine the association (correlational analysis) between self-report of memory difficulties and performance on a test of memory. High correlations would help to establish concurrent validity. One caveat is that if patients were to rate their memory impairment following their actual test performance, the relationships might be spurious. In other words, patients who are depressed often have negative self-appraisals and assume that they did poorly on memory tests despite occasional "normal" performance. On the other hand, patients who perform poorly on memory testing may be well aware that they did not do well on testing, and they may then rate their perception of their memory performance accordingly. Therefore, it is preferred that the test score and outcome measure are obtained from different sources (e.g., a patient and his or her spouse).

Concurrent validity would be more useful with two modality-congruent tests (e.g., two memory tests) rather than mixing and matching the methods of assessment (performance and observer report). The correlations among measures of similar methodologies are likely to be more reliable and valid.

Predictive Validity

As the name suggests, predictive validity establishes how well a particular variable predicts a criterion variable. In this case, the temporal relationship between the test score (which is assessed first) and the outcome measure (assessed last) is essential in order for the researcher to aver that one predicts another. Again, it is not the same to say that a score that precedes a particular outcome caused the outcome. In fact, as Anastasi (1950) argued over 60 years ago, a psychological test is simply a device for determining within a brief period what would eventually emerge with time. For example, we could say that performance on an intelligence test at age 12 predicts whether this person will pursue graduate training. However, the outcome measure (whether or not this person is to pursue graduate training) will reveal itself in due time. Thus, neuropsychological tests are useful in that they provide such predictions of important outcomes, be they academic or medical, well in advance of such protracted observations (Anastasi, 1950).

Using informant ratings of patients' behavior as a predictor of patients developing frontotemporal dementia later in life would be an example of establishing a test's predictive validity. The test score—the informant's report—is culled prior to the criterion (diagnosis of a disease). The method of analysis appropriate for this example would be logistic regression, where the outcome measure is dichotomous (a person does or does not develop the disease). The allure of logistic regression is that it provides both the classification accuracy of the model (how many people who were rated as having behavior difficulties are actually diagnosed with frontotemporal dementia), as well as odds ratios. Odds ratios allow for the examination of an increase or decrease in odds of developing the disease based on informant ratings for every unit increase on the behavior rating scale.

The criterion variable need not be categorical. For example, one can use a scale of postpartum depression to examine levels (gradations) of depression years later (of course, with appropriate covariates in the model). This would involve a multiple regression analysis.

The use of regression models (either linear or logistic) in establishing predictive validity also allows the researcher to explore the contributions of other factors, as well as control for other relevant and possibly confounding factors.

Construct Validity

The construct validity of a measure is another way of verifying the relationship between a particular measure and the concept it purportedly gauges. An instrument should operate systematically and in accord with an underlying construct. That is, persons who are inherently high on a particular skill or trait should perform accordingly on a test of this particular ability. Neuropsychological measures are proxies for neuropsychological constructs; these measures should be considered operational definitions of these very constructs. As mentioned earlier, an operational definition is an explicit, quantifiable definition of the inclusion and exclusion criteria of a construct. For example, in developing a scale for aggression, researchers must decide whether to include verbal, physical, and/or passive aggressiveness into their definition. Once this is determined, the scale should assess only the relevant parameters of this construct.

As Bryant (2000) notes, face validity is somewhat related to construct validity, as it concerns the degree to which a measure appears to assess what it is intended. The immediate and delayed recall of information, for example, can be quite readily viewed as measures of learning and memory.

On the other hand, alternating between encircled numbers and letters on the Trail Making Test may not be such an obvious measure of executive cognition. Empirically, though, the Trail Making Test has been substantiated as a quite robust test of executive cognition. Similarly, self-ratings on the personality assessment inventory (PAI) (Morey, 1991) may be unrevealing to the naked eye. However, several items on the PAI tap peculiar and perhaps unlikely experiences that may suggest a psychogenic rather than an organic problem. However, the intent of these items is not (and should not be) apparent, and patients are generally unaware that clinically relevant (e.g., malingering versus psychosis) information is trying to be gleaned.

There are two broad criteria for assessing the construct validity of an instrument: convergent and divergent validity. The purpose of using such measures, often in combination, is to establish the specificity of a construct. Separate scales that tap into the same construct should be equally influenced. On the other hand, instruments that have no conceptual relation with a construct should not bear any statistical association.

Convergent Validity

Convergent validity examines whether instruments assessing the same construct "converge," or are in agreement. This merely means that if two measures are assessing the same underlying concept, they should behave similarly, and this evidently should manifest as a high correlation between the two instruments. For example, if performance on a test of activities of daily living (e.g., texas functional living scale; TFLS) (Cullum, Weiner, & Saine, 2009) is indeed an ecologically valid measure (i.e., samples a person's ability (or lack thereof) to perform similar activities out of the testing room), it should correlate highly with other valid measures: informant ratings of the person's activities of daily living; the number of errors they made cooking a meal at home, etc.

In developing a test of auditory/verbal learning and memory, high correlations should be demonstrated with other ("gold standards") tests that measure identical functions (e.g., Hopkins Verbal Learning Test—Revised) (Brandt & Benedict, 2001). High correlations between the two tests signify that these measures are presumably tapping into a unique dimension of cognition.

Divergent Validity

Divergent validity assesses whether measures of dissimilar constructs "diverge," in that they show no obvious relationship. This ensures both the integrity and the specificity of a construct.

If a new scale or depression was significantly related to another test of depression in a bivariate correlation, but this scale was completely distinct (uncorrelated) with a scale assessing anxiety, this would establish the test's divergent validity (as well as its convergent validity, since it is also correlated with another scale of depression).

Factor-analytic methods are common techniques for examining a measure's convergent and divergent validity simultaneously. Factor analysis, as discussed in this book, examines the covariation among a large number of items. Items that are highly correlated are subsumed under a particular factor, as they are assumed to be assessing the same latent variable or hypothetical construct. For example, to ensure the construct validity of a new instrument measuring a distinct component of depression, say social withdrawal, all individual items from this scale would be entered into the analysis. To corroborate social withdrawal's construct validity (i.e., construct validation), all items that relate to social withdrawal (e.g., preferring to stay at home rather than venture out, etc.) should load onto one factor. This establishes the convergent validity of the measure. On the other hand, if other items that tap into anhedonia and physiological symptoms of depression loaded separately, representing a distinct dimension of affective symptoms, this would provide evidence for social withdrawal's divergent validity. Together, the construct's convergent and divergent validity coalesce to establish construct validity.

There are other ways of determining a measure's divergent validity, such as simple bivariate correlations between measures. However, as convergent and divergent validity are often assessed concurrently, multivariate procedures are often preferred (e.g., Campbell & Fisk, 1959).

Clinical Validation

Bryant (2000) also discussed clinical validation in which researchers evaluate the accuracy with which scores on a given instrument can classify groups that are already known to differ on a criterion measure. For example, logistic regression analysis could be implemented to determine whether a screen for cognitive impairment differentiates persons with mild cognitive impairment and those healthy elderly persons (patients and healthy elderly persons represent the dichotomous criterion variable in the logistic regression analysis). This is clearly a subset of criterion validity, but it earns its moniker from the clinical context in which the data analysis arises.

Incremental Validity

Incremental validity holds a special place within clinical neuropsychology. The main goal of incremental validity is to determine whether the addition of potentially clinically relevant variables (e.g., test performance) contributes to a particular criterion measure over and above traditional tests. Statistically, this method involves examining the change in the proportion of variance explained in the dependent variable with the inclusion of an additional predictor. This is generally couched within a hierarchical regression analysis with the variable of primary importance placed in the last block (see chapter on regression).

It is important in neuropsychology to demonstrate that measures are able to improve classification or prediction above and beyond typical tests or measures used for diagnosis. This is exactly what we are looking at with incremental validity—how much more variance does a test, index, instrument explain *above and beyond* what is explained by other tests. More specifically, does a new test or measure improve an outcome measure beyond traditional tests? Does adding this measure help explain an outcome variable more so than if it had not been included?

As mentioned, hierarchical regression analysis is a commonly used method for examining the incremental validity of a test or measure. This holds true for either logistic regression (when you are classifying a binary outcome, such as normal controls and patients) or linear regression (when the outcome variable is continuous).

Busch, Frazier, Haggerty, and Kubu (2005) explored performance on the Boston Naming Test among 217 patients with intractable temporal lobe epilepsy (all right handed; 108 with left temporal lobe epilepsy and 109 with right temporal lobe epilepsy) and its ability to predict the ultimate side of surgery above and beyond the ability of indices of intellectual function (Verbal Comprehension Index and Perceptual Organization Index from the WAIS-III). In the hierarchical logistic regression analysis, scores from the WAIS-III along with a measure of delayed memory were entered into block/step 1. The raw score from the Boston Naming test was entered in block two. The dependent variable was the side of surgery (i.e., left or right).

To determine the significance of this model, the authors examined the last step (Step 2) to determine whether the raw score from the Boston Naming Test was significant. These authors examined the change in R^2 (proportion of variance) from models one (with just the scores from intelligence and memory) to model two (with the Boston Naming Test) to determine if this was a significant change in the prediction of side of surgery. The final model was significant, which supports the incremental validity of using the Boston Naming Test in classifying right versus left hemisphere surgery (among these particular tests).

Ecological Validity

Ecological validity has to do with how well neuropsychological tests are both conceptually and empirically related with activities of daily living (e.g., paying bills, driving, managing finances and medicines, misplacing one's keys, etc.).

Chaytor and Schmitter-Edgecombe (2003) recount the advent of technological advances (e.g., brain imaging) that have replaced certain goals of neuropsychological assessment. Brain imaging has supplanted neuropsychology from a practice of corroborating brain pathology (in most cases) to more broad applications that typically include the functioning of a person in whom pathology has been documented. Neuropsychologists are generally not counseled to opine on the mere presence of an organic etiology. This shift in roles for neuropsychology has required the profession to accommodate to an ever-changing environment. Simply put, brain imaging (whether structural or functional) will reveal nothing about a person's cognitive, behavioral, emotional, or functional capacities.

Chaytor and Schmitter-Edgecombe (2003) discuss two conceptual principles for establishing ecological validity: verisimilitude and veridicality. Verisimilitude concerns the correspondence and equivalency of tests and real-world demands. For example, tests are developed to simulate every day activities, such as writing a check, or using a telephone. Veridicality involves the degree to which a test shows an empirical relation to measures of everyday functioning (Franzen & Wilhelm, 1996). For example, a performance-based measure of daily activities—the texas functional living scale (TFLS) (Cullum et al., 2009)—should demonstrate a strong association with other aspects of real-world abilities, such as employment, or informant reports of the patient's activities of daily living.

Neuropsychological assessment remains weak at capturing all aspects that contribute to an individual's ability to function in the real world. There is a clear dissociation between a patient's performance on testing, and what he or she can do in his daily life. For one, unlike the real world, testing entails a distraction free, structured setting. There are also a host of noncognitive or nonintellectual factors that contribute to daily functioning. For example, personality and emotional difficulties, physical and sensory limitations, availability to certain resources (financial and environmental), living situations (e.g., house, apartment, dependence on car or public transportation, etc.) and many other perhaps ineffable factors affect, either for the better or worse, daily functioning (Chaytor & Schmitter-Edgecombe, 2003).

Summary

This chapter discussed validity as it pertains to neuropsychology. Five principal aspects of validity were delineated: Content, criterion, construct, incremental, and ecological. Such methods vary in their conceptual and practical goals, but show considerable overlap in terms of the statistical models that attempt to establish their veracity.

Whereas content validity ensures that the items used on a test are theoretically culled from a population of relevant items to ensure exhaustiveness in its assessment, methods for criterion validity (postdictive, concurrent, and predictive) vary predominantly in the temporal order in which the variables are assessed. The goal of criterion validity is to ensure that tests we use as proxies for certain behaviors are associated, and presumably, can predict a future outcome. Construct validity (convergent and divergent) ensures that the constructs we use in neuropsychology are indeed evaluating what we say they are. Incremental validity helps improve prediction of additional tests and constructs by demonstrating their unique contribution to classifying particular outcomes over and above standard methods. And, ecological validity attempts to bridge the gap between what is exhibited on neuropsychological testing and what is experienced in the real world. That is, how well does performance on neuropsychological testing reflect one's daily functioning? Does someone who has trouble with various activities of daily living show commensurate difficulty when examined in an office by a neuropsychologist?

Overall, validity is a process of establishing a test's clinical utility in describing, explaining, and predicting phenomena. Validity is not a function of a test per se, but is inextricably entwined with the context in which a test is applied.

Chapter 3
Assumptions of Statistical Analyses

Surveying the Damage: Searching for Discrepancies in Data Entry and Ensuring the Appropriate Application of Statistical Analyses

Once data are accessible, it is quite tempting to run the main analysis. Nowadays, analyzing data is effortless: all one needs is a few spare minutes. However, as enticing as this is, there are many things you might want to consider before running the analysis (or analyses), including checking for errors in data entry and deciding what to do with missing values and outliers (extreme scores).

There are a number of references for detecting and dealing with outliers, handling missing data, as well as a host of other data management issues. These problems should be considered before any type of main analysis is run. They are beyond the scope of this book.

The next step in data analysis—before the actual, data analysis in most cases—involves examination of statistical assumptions. The data must assume essential characteristics so that the models we use to overlay on the observed data do not mislead us and/or misinform us or both. This chapter will telescope its discussion to the more common assumption's in statistical analyses.

Statistical Assumptions

An assumption, as you are well aware, is a supposition, something that we take for granted, a belief that we hold about something (e.g., an event) that can range from the very likely to the likely improbable: your hot water will be working in the morning so that you can take a shower; how much money you will earn after graduating from college; that purchasing this book would be worth your while. A *statistical* assumption means that we presume that our data take on particular characteristics

D.A. Maroof, *Statistical Methods in Neuropsychology: Common Procedures Made Comprehensible*, DOI 10.1007/978-1-4614-3417-7_3,

(e.g., that the data are normally distributed), or that the way in which data are collected (including how participants are selected) was done so accurately (e.g., independence of observations; to be discussed shortly), so that the application of certain statistical tests [t-tests, analysis of variance (ANOVA)] is unbiased, and so that researchers can be confident that their interpretations, and ultimately, their inferences, are robust and reliable.

Examining assumptions before engaging in any activity may be time consuming, but can prove for a better outcome and experience. Let us say you were to assume that a store was still open at 9 PM. You grab your keys, slip on your shoes, drive 20 min, weather the DJ's horrific selection of music—as if he were implicitly mocking those who were unfortunate enough to be out in their cars at this time of night on a weekday—but the store is closed. The next time you decide to venture out to the store at night, you call ahead to ensure that they are open and will remain open for the next hour or so. In this case, whether they are open or closed benefits you: if they are closed you just saved yourself about 40 min of travel time, gas, and exposure to lousy music. If open, you get to go to the store and buy yourself a new copy of your new favorite author's book (please, I'm blushing).

Starting to sink in? We are to apply this same logic to our data. Before we "go out to the store" (analyze and interpret our data), we call first. We must ensure that our methods for collecting data and the distributions of these data assume certain characteristics.

There are two general ways of examining assumptions: methodologically and statistically/analytically. Methodologically, one can "build in" to a study certain parameters (e.g., the constitution of the population we are to examine; matching, etc.). The analytic (statistical) method includes graphical and/or statistical means for exploring the distribution of data (e.g., are the data normally distributed?; Shapiro–Wilk test: are the variances between or among groups disparate?; Levene's test). I will review core assumptions and some more "advanced" assumptions as they pertain to particular data-analytic procedures.

What Are the Most Common Statistical Assumptions?

Although there are a substantial number of statistical tests, several rely on core assumptions. I will review a good many here. Keep in mind that although assumptions should be examined prior to running the primary analyses, as violations of these assumptions often render inaccurate the results from standard parametric tests, certain methods of examining assumptions require the analysis be executed first (e.g., residual analysis).

Another simple tip: interpreting the significance of assumptions often runs counter to what we look for when interpreting our main analyses. That is, we generally *do not* want the tests of assumptions to be statistically significant, as this indicates that our assumption has been violated (e.g., if Levene's test were significant, it means that the variances between two groups are different), rendering our inferences/interpretations untenable or suspect. On the other hand, we often hope that the results from the main analyses (e.g., comparing the difference between group means) *are* significant. In this case, we can say that there exists a significant difference, with hopes that this is in line with the a priori hypothesis!

Independence of Observations

Aptly named. Let us say that I was to administer a list-learning task (e.g., Hopkins Verbal Learning Test—Revised; HVLT-R) (Brandt & Benedict, 2001) to a group, rather than to an individual. I read aloud all the items on the list, and then have each person, one-by-one, say aloud the words that they could recall. To get to the point, after the first individual utters what he recalls, the next person can recall not only the words he recalls from the examiner's presentation but also each consecutive participant's performance will be enhanced (at least, they have the opportunity to benefit) from hearing the list recited again and again by the preceding participants. Therefore, we say that the observations, or the data (i.e., how many words are recalled), are not independent. Rather, they are dependent on the methodology used for data collection, that is, on other persons' responses.

There are also several self-administered questionnaires we use in neuropsychology. Perhaps we were interested in quantifying a person's depressive symptoms/severity of depression by use of the Beck Depression Inventory (BDI) (Beck, Ward, Mendelson, Mock, & Erbaugh, 1961). Instead of having the person sit by himself to complete the BDI, we ask him each question in front of his spouse or his parents. Let us say that this individual is quite depressed, and although willing to acknowledge this to a mental health professional, he is loath to do so in front of his family. Therefore, he purposefully forswears certain, if not all, questions that would suggest depression, including hopelessness. This is not only a horrible thing to do from a clinical standpoint in that we might be conveying to the patient that we are more interested in the data we receive rather than what these data are intended to measure. From a statistical point of view, this practice makes for *dependence* of observations. This person's responses to the BDI are dependent, or contingent, upon the presence of his family.

Violation of the assumption of independence of observations is circumvented by methodological design. There is no way to overcome such a fatal flaw with fancy statistical techniques such as covarying for nuisance variables. We ensure that the scores among participants are not dependent on one another by building this into how the data are collected. This is such a crucial statistical assumption, and is such standard practice in experimental design, that authors rarely if ever make mention of satisfying it.

Normality

Normally (get it?), it is assumed that most, but not all, variables assume a bell-shaped, Gaussian, distribution. In other words, if I selected a sample of participants, I would assume that perhaps their education or age would be normally distributed. Not everyone would have the exact level of education—some completed high school, others college, still others with graduate-level training. However, we might assume that most people in our sample are high school or college graduates. We would expect that there are far fewer persons with higher (Master's level or doctorate) or much lower (with only an elementary school education) education. Why? Because these data points are extreme values. The majority of people do not drop out of school in the 2nd grade, nor do most people we know (in general) earn doctoral degrees. If these values were plotted on a graph, it would assume a normal distribution. Most people pile up around high school/college level education, whereas, the tails of the distribution reflect the many fewer persons who fall into the extremes. From a clinical standpoint, scores that fall into the extremes are ways in which we determine whether a person's performance on any given measure is "abnormally" low or high (i.e., deficient or superior, respectively).

Similarly, age varies. Some people selected for study may be in their 20s, others in their 30s, and so on. So, some are young, some middle-aged, and some old—or just older. However, in these "theoretical" distributions, the percentage of individuals that represent each age band differ. In other words, it is a mathematical given that about 68% of the population will fall anywhere from one standard deviation below the mean to one standard deviation above the mean. About 95% of the population fall between two standard deviations below the mean to two standard deviations above the mean. Clearly, as the range of scores is expanded, the percentage of the population that fall within that very range increase as well, since you will be including more and more of the population. Also notice that a larger percentage of persons fall within ranges closer to the mean. A smaller percentage of people represent the same range of standard deviation units in the tail ends of the distribution. This is because the larger number of persons by mathematical necessity hover around the mean.

Unfortunately, many neuropsychological tests do not take on normal distributions (Brooks, Strauss, Sherman, Iverson, & Slick, 2009). Common examples include the Boston Naming Test and the Wisconsin Card Sorting Test (Strauss, Sherman, & Spreen, 2006). Most persons without neurologic illness are able to name most, if not all, line-drawn objects on the Boston Naming Test. The result: a negatively skewed distribution. There are ways of outwitting these distributions in clinical decision-making and statistical analysis, including inspection of cumulative percentages.

Although most studies do not report the results of whether their data did or did not violate statistical assumptions, it is a good idea to get in the habit of assessing these assumptions and informing your reader that you have done so, prior to the bulk of your data analysis. Whether you examine, report, and respond appropriately to the results of these explorations, this can ultimately affect the precision of the results, and therefore, the integrity of your interpretations.

Homogeneity of Variance

Variance is another term for difference, or dispersion. So, this means that the dispersion or variability of scores among groups of participants derive from populations with similar variances. Again, there are inferential tests to tell us whether this might be a problem (e.g., Levene's Test). If this test is significant, then we have violated this assumption.

As an example, a group of patients with schizophrenia and normal control participants are administered an intelligence test. It could be theorized that the healthy participants should have for the most part IQs that are roughly average. Therefore, some may be somewhat above average, and some below. The variability about the mean is negligible. In contrast, patients with schizophrenia may show considerable variability on an intelligence test. First, patients may have acquired limited knowledge because their illness interfered with its acquisition, rendering their performance below average. There may be some patients who were functioning very well, and tackle the test without much effort. Although I am merely telling stories, the point is that these patients may show more variability than the healthy participants, and the variances between the groups may be significantly different. This variability creates a small signal to noise ratio, making any veritable differences between groups indiscernible.

Homoscedasticity

This assumption pertains to regression, but it is an important one so it's discussed here. A good example of violating homoscedasticity (referred to as heteroscedasticity) would be your commute to work. Let us say the time you left in the morning was the independent variable, and the dependent variable was how long it took you to arrive to work. If you leave anywhere between 4 AM and 7 AM, you arrive to work within 35 min. If you leave between 7 AM and 8:30 AM, your average travel time to work is 55 min. If you leave between 9 AM and 9:30 AM, it may take you an hour and 20 min. (If you leave around 10 AM or later, you may miss the morning traffic, and it may take you less time to arrive at work.) The amount of traffic, and the time it takes you to get to work, varies as a function of when you leave for work. So, we see that the variability of driving time to work—the error—differs as a function of our independent variable (when we leave). Therefore, if we tried to apply a linear model to these data assuming that the later you leave for work, the longer it takes (which might be assumed based on truncated data, i.e., examining the pattern between only 4 AM and 9:30 AM), it might not be appropriate (unless we transform that data) because of a potential violation of homoscedasticity.

Let us use this example within the context of neuropsychology. Hypothetically, if we were to examine something as simple as learning as a function of age in a group of normal persons, individuals who range in age from 20 through 55 were intact, and generally performed very close to the ceiling on list learning tests. However, individuals above 55, perhaps because of early onset neurodegenerative illness, vascular illness that commonly results in slowed information processing speed, the scores are more variable. Thus, the persons in the older age ranges show marked variability. Some perform poorly, some at the normal range, and some well above average. What we need to explore prior to examining say a linear relationship between age and memory, is whether we are encountering heteroscedasticity; the variance (difference) of the error term is *not* constant across different levels of the independent (age) variable.

Studies that Have Used and Reported Assumptions

It is all too common that research articles make no mention of assumptions. Either examining assumptions is too effortful, or assumptions are just not considered important. Some researchers may report it. For example, take this paragraph from a recent article that examined object naming errors among subgroups of primary progressive aphasia and one post-stroke (left hemisphere) group (Budd, Kortte, Cloutman, Newhart, Gottesman, et al., 2010; pg. 584):

> *Before conducting the main analyses, data from naming tests and subject data were tested for normality, linearity, and the presence of outliers. Additionally, identification of potential confounding variables (potential group differences on age, education, and naming error rate) was undertaken by conducting a series of ANOVAs...Bonferonni correction for multiple comparisons was applied.*

The paragraph above informs the reader that assumptions of their statistical analyses were not only under consideration, but also were examined prior to their main analyses. And a simple tip, most readers prefer the laconic to the prolix. There is no need to provide excessive detail. If something you feel is salient, mention it. If you are correcting your data because of an assumption violation, tell the reader *briefly* how you did so, and *why* you chose a particular method over another.

Summary

Now you should have a basic understanding of some common statistical assumptions. There are a number of methods for managing violations (transformations of data, using nonparametric instead of parametric tests), which are highly recommended. Meeting assumptions is an important part of statistical analysis, and should be handled appropriately. It is unwise to simply ride roughshod over such fundamental principles that can skew the results and any subsequent interpretations.

Chapter 4
Exploratory Factor Analysis

An Introduction

Exploratory factor analysis (EFA) helps establish the bedrock of how neuropsychologists interpret the tests used in their evaluative process. Its principle goal concerns the reification of abstract psychological and neuropsychological concepts. Thus, recall of designs or a lengthy word list materializes to visual and verbal memory, respectively.

EFA aids in defining and discriminating neuropsychological constructs: memory, attention, language, executive function, and spatial cognition. These constructs, in turn, help depict the cognitive "footprint" of various neurologic disorders, infer the neural substrates implicated in suspected illness, and correlate known neurologic lesions and disease processes to their cognitive, behavioral, and emotional expressions.

The overarching goal of EFA is to make sense of the large number of cognitive tests administered and/or the spate of scores and indices generated from any one neuropsychological test battery. The data must transform into a more manageable and economical solution. EFA helps accomplish this goal by harnessing and condensing information from multiple tests—or countless scores from one test.

The objective of EFA is to supplant individual scores with constructs/factors that *embody* the content *and* intentions of the original/individual test items. These constructs are used descriptively (e.g., as when we say a patient's performance on a test of *memory* is poor) and inferentially (e.g., as when we say that based on a patient's poor test performances, his or her *memory* is impaired) Constructs, and the test scores they represent, serve as yardsticks for neuropsychological functioning.

The constructs generated and retained in EFA reflect the variation and covariation of responses and performances on testing. Items that are highly correlated are clustered together. Each band of correlated scores is assumed to invoke a distinct cognitive process, or affective or behavioral state. Ultimately, each collection of related items is subsumed under the rubric of one particular factor, representing a

D.A. Maroof, *Statistical Methods in Neuropsychology: Common Procedures Made Comprehensible*, DOI 10.1007/978-1-4614-3417-7_4,

latent variable. Interestingly, whereas most multivariate statistics involve well-defined independent and dependent variables, EFA analyzes a number of items or test scores and "generates" factor scores (variables in their own right).

The purpose of this chapter is to describe the most common applications of EFA. The steps involved in choosing to run and interpret an EFA are broken down. A very simple illustration of data often analyzed in factor analysis and how factors are interpreted and "labeled" is provided.

What Exactly Does EFA Do?

EFA examines patterns of interrelationships among data, serving to winnow down the range of explanatory phenomena from a large number of test scores for further classification, description, and clarity.

We use test scores as proxies for brain function; these scores should vary within and across measures if they are indeed measuring similar and dissimilar brain functions, respectively. EFA seeks concision by examining how many—or how few—factors underlie a large number of items.

EFA is a prime example of a statistical technique that epitomizes one very central psychological principle: parsimony. For example, the purpose of administering a 567-item self-administered inventory (i.e., the Minnesota Multiphasic Personality Inventory-2; MMPI-2) (Butcher, Graham, Ben-Porath, Tellegen, Dahlstrom, & Kaemmer, 2001) is *not* to generate a list of 567 adjectives to describe a person. The purpose, rather, is to provide an abbreviated and concentrated narrative of an individual. This is why the MMPI-2 along with other self-administered inventories (e.g., Personality Assessment Inventory; PAI) (Morey, 1991) yields scales (e.g., Depression). Based on a person's responses, these scales (which comprise a number of conceptually related items) are systematically influenced. If someone responds to items that reflect depression, then the scale for depression will (should) be elevated accordingly, providing clinically relevant, and easily identifiable, information. At times, of course, some information may be overlooked. For example, focusing on the construct of depression does not necessarily inform the clinician of the specific symptoms: whether the person is helpless, hopeless, or suicidal, for example. As such, in clinical practice it is wise to examine each item qualitatively when there is an elevation.

To underscore and reiterate, constructs provide conceptually broad, yet succinct clinical information. It is easier and more practical to describe someone as "dependable" rather than providing a list of behaviors that comprise the concept/construct of "dependability": "he regularly shows up to work on time," "he calls when he says he will," "his work is always done on time." To minimize verbiage, it is equally common to condense information, such as labeling someone as unkempt, rather than discussing his or her hygiene and comportment ad nauseum. Likewise, the purpose of administering a lengthy list-learning test is not to describe how many and which

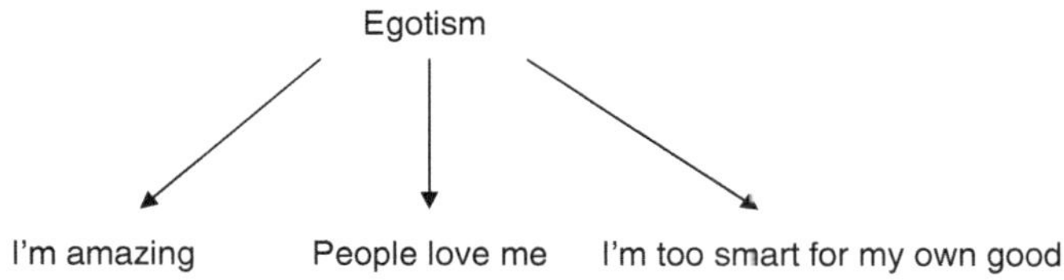

Fig. 4.1 Individual test items that are aspects of the construct, "egotism"

items they recalled; this would be uninformative. However, to infer that someone performed poorly on all tests that assess learning and memory speaks volumes.

For the reasons I described above, it is no wonder EFA is considered a data reduction procedure: a large number of items (e.g., test scores) are clumped together to form distinct constructs (factors). These factors form the linchpin of conceptual reasoning and clinical decision making, as we infer the integrity of an ability, or the degree of a syndrome (e.g., depression), by examining test performance and item endorsement, respectively. Statistically, EFA assesses the variation and covariation among a large number of both related and unrelated items. Based on tests' or items' peaks and troughs, and examining which do so in unison, we can deduce a neuropsychological theme underlying a set of items.

EFA is also used when trying to establish a measure's construct validity: whether a test is measuring what we think it's measuring. In the development or evaluation of tests believed to assess certain cognitive abilities—processing speed, memory, and intelligence—inchoate tests are benchmarked against existing and validated tests. Establishing that these emergent tests purportedly measure a similar cognitive function with conventional tests of that very same cognitive, based on their correlations, marshals further evidence that what makes these tests fluctuate together is likely a shared fundamental dimension of human affect, cognition or behavior.

As shown in Fig. 4.1, the construct of "egotism" might comprise samples of one's thoughts.

The Organization of Neuropsychological Constructs

Factors can be organized across or within constructs. "Across constructs" measure conceptually disparate aspects of human experience: memory, language, executive function, anxiety, etc. On the other hand, factors that are organized "within constructs" signify varying levels of an operational definition's specificity. For example, subsumed under the rubric of memory can lie immediate recall, delayed recall, and recognition. Similarly, cognitive function may be represented by separate modes of cognitive faculty (see Figs. 4.2 and 4.3).

Fig. 4.2 Organization of the construct of depression (Within construct specificity)

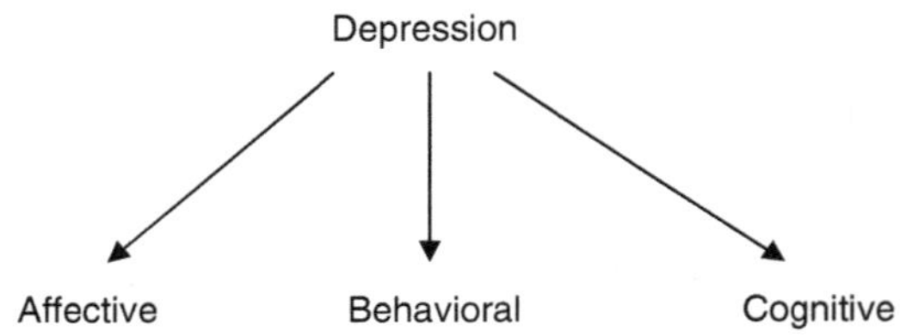

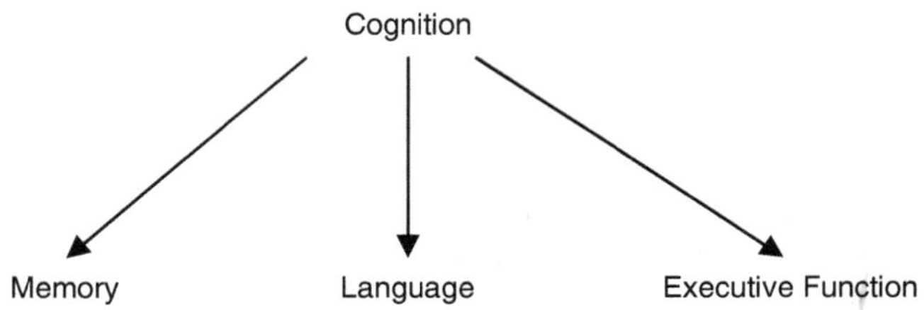

Fig. 4.3 Organization of the construct of cognition (Across construct specificity)

Purposes of EFA

EFA serves a few general purposes (DeVellis, 2003). Ultimately, EFA explores the number of categories that are sufficient to summarize the majority of information contained in the original set of items. Unfortunately, it is inevitable that some of the original information is diluted and lost in translation. However, the benefits overall outweigh the costs. The purposes of EFA (according to DeVellis, 2003) include the following:

1. How many latent variables (constructs) underlie a set of items/responses; or how few factors can characterize the set of test items without losing much of the original information derived from the individual test items
2. Condensation: to explain variation among several variables using far fewer newly created variables
3. To define meaning/classification of the factors that account for variation among the items. Items/tests should serve as "signposts" that inform and guide one to a common underlying theme (factor). Items may reflect learning and memory, speed of processing, depression, disinhibition, apathy, etc.

What Are Some Assumptions of EFA?

EFA assumes that several latent constructs underlie multiple measures or scores. EFA *does not* assume that only one latent variable is the source of all variation among the test items.

Cronbach's alpha (Cronbach, 1951) is a measure of internal test reliability, and is predicated on the assumption that all test items reflect only one underlying construct. One can therefore think of EFA as an extension of Cronbach's alpha (although it is not a test of validity, but reliability), much as we can think of multiple regression as an extension of simple linear regression, or of multivariate analysis of variance as an extension of an univariate analysis of variance.

If one were to examine an index of anxiety that assesses physiological (e.g., tachycardia, sweaty palms), cognitive ("If I go to the store, I am likely to have a panic attack"), and behavioral (e.g., social withdrawal) features, a Cronbach's alpha may not be appropriate given that this particular concept of anxiety reflects various levels of specificity. Presumably, one could calculate Cronbach's alpha on each set of questions that pertain to each one of these three aspects of anxiety. However, it would be more sensible to run an EFA; three factors that explain the majority of the variation among items should emerge.

What Are the Steps for EFA?

EFA is an iterative process, and involves the following four steps (Ford, MacCallum, & Tait, 1986):

1. Choosing the model
2. Selecting/extracting factors to retain
3. Applying rotation methods
4. Interpretation of the factor solution

Choosing the Model

One must determine whether EFA is appropriate for the question (s) being asked. This must also be determined based on other factors: how many participants does one have access to and how many items are available. Generally, there is a proposed subject-to-item ratio—10:1which is the prevalent rule-of-thumb for determining an adequate sample size (Costello & Osborne, 2005).

A crucial step in the process is also deciding on which of the items available should be included in the analysis. Although EFA is essentially a hypothesis seeking procedure rather than a hypothesis testing procedure, it is still unwise to select tests merely because they are available. Although it is not uncommon to deselect a few items should they have very small factor loadings after a preliminary exploration of the data. However, minor modifications to item inclusion can drastically change the resultant factor structure, rendering the results spurious and sample specific.

A crucial step in this process of EFA entails choosing a factor extraction method (e.g., unweighted least squares, maximum likelihood, principal axis factoring, etc.).

Programs such as SPSS have principal components analysis as the default method. Although beyond the scope of this chapter, the extraction method best suited for analysis generally hinges on the distribution of the data. For example, maximum likelihood is best suited when the data are normally distributed (Costello & Osborne, 2005).

Extracting Factors

Extraction is an iterative process. The extraction method produces factor loadings for every item on every extracted factor. These factor loadings are essentially the correlations between the individual items/scores and the latent factor. As the latent variable is unobservable (it is a creation from the relationships among all variables in a particular factor), these factor loadings represent the estimated relationship between the observable correlations and the latent construct.

The hope of EFA is to disclose *simple structure*—most items having large loadings on one factor, but small loadings on other factors. If a variable has high loadings on more than on dimension, they may need to be discarded. And, the sign (positive or negative), of the coefficient reveals whether the item is directly or inversely related with the construct, respectively.

The procedure presupposes that only one construct can explain the variation among all of the scores. However, if one concept/construct is inadequate in accounting for the covariation among the items, then, the model proceeds with extracting the residual item covariation. This continues until the variance explained that the model has not accounted for is negligible. As DeVellis (2003) notes, the data analyst appraises the amount of information each successive factor contains and judges when a point of "diminishing returns" has been reached.

Unlike other factor analytic methods (e.g., confirmatory factor analysis) that require statistical criteria for model fit and significance, EFA has been criticized for its seemingly subjective nature. For example, a very common method for determining how many factors to retain involves examining the percentage of variance in the variables that is accounted for by the factor. Generally, the factors should explain at least 50% of the variation and covariation among the variables.

The two more common "nonstatistical" methods for factor extraction include: the eigenvalue rule (Kaiser, 1960) and the scree test (Catell, 1966). The goal of these two procedures is to establish how a few factors shoulder the most influential sources of variation underlying the set of items. These methods are at times used in isolation, but clinicians and researchers are encouraged to use both (if not multiple) methods for factor extraction (Fabrigar, Wegener, MacCallum, & Strahan, 1999). There are other measures of factor retention, including Velicer's MAP (Minimum Average Partial) criteria (Velicer & Jackson, 1990), and parallel analysis (Hayton, Allen, & Scarpello, 2004).

Hayton et al. (2004) provide a step-by-step explanation of calculating parallel analysis, which they note attempts to overcome one of the primary limitations of Kaiser's greater-than-one eigenvalue rule by adjusting for the effects of sampling error, thereby reducing the possibility of spurious factors.

Eigenvalue Rule

An eigenvalue (Kaiser, 1960) represents the amount of information captured by a factor, or in other words, the variance accounted for by each underlying factor. Eigenvalues are not represented by percentages but discrete values (e.g., 1, 2, etc.) that total the number of items in the analysis. Technically, the number of factors can equal the number of items included in the analysis. Each factor will have an eigenvalue that indicates the amount of variation in the items accounted for by each factor. Although calculated in statistical software packages (e.g., SPSS), the percentage of variance explained for each factor can be calculated by dividing the eigenvalue (e.g., 1, 2, 3, etc.) by the total number of items in the analysis; the larger the eigenvalue, the more information contained in any given factor. So, if the first factor has an eigenvalue of 5, and 20 items were analyzed, this factor captures 25% of the total variance ($5/20 \times 100 = 25\%$). The first factor always secures the greatest amount variance, as this is an iterative process wherein the first factor "usurps" all of the common variation.

Based on the value of eigenvalues, researchers decide on whether the factor it represents warrants inclusion in the final model. High eigenvalues (e.g., greater than 1) indicate that a factor captures an adequate portion of variance (Guttman, 1954) and should be considered for retention. Eigenvalues less than 1 signify that a factor captures less variance than any common item and should not be considered for retention. In fact the eigenvalues with low values are likely to be describing error variance, or to be representing influences that affect only one or a few of the test items (Harris, 2001).

Although not generally used in practice, some have argued (Larsen & Warne, 2010) that because eigenvalues are point estimates, it is more appropriate to calculate confidence intervals for the eigenvalues. Some reasons for doing so include the fact that the American Psychiatric Association (APA) mandates that such statistics are provided for sample statistics (which eigenvalues are), and because confidence intervals provide more information to the reader and increase transparency in EFA research. Another reason for including confidence intervals is to serve as an enhancement to traditional methods of deciding the number of factors to retain.

Table 4.1 shows a selected amount of information commonly generated in computer software.

Scree Plot/Test

Scree is a term used for any disintegrated material, or rubble, on the side of a mountain. The "scree" that this test is referring to is the inconsequential eigenvalues (e.g., less than one), which should not be considered for inclusion in the final factor model. The scree test (Catell, 1966) is somewhat like a visual analogue to the eigenvalue test. However,

Table 4.1 Principal components analysis—selected output

Component	Eigenvalues total	Eigenvalues % variance	Cum. % variance
1	3.2	35.6	35.6
2	1.2	13.4	49.0
3	1.0	11.5	60.5
4	0.93	10.4	70.8
5	0.74	8.2	79.0
6	0.66	7.4	86.4
7	0.58	6.5	92.8

the resultant factor structure relies more on a qualitative, relative methodology as opposed to the eigenvalue method, which relies on the absolute, numerical value (e.g., generally greater than 1.0) (DeVellis, 2003).

The scree test is a plot of the eigenvalues (on the ordinate, or y-axis) and the factors (on the abscissa, or x-axis). Based on what was discussed earlier, each subsequent factor is the residual from the previous extraction, and thus, will always be less than any prior eigenvalue.

In order to determine how many factors to retain, the relative drop in eigenvalues, referred to as the elbow, is "eye-balled." There is often a precipitous drop, and then a sudden shift into a plateau in the horizontal plane. Generally, the number of factors retained lies in the vertical portion of the graph (but not at the point at which the plateau begins). The smaller eigenvalues to the right are not substantive (the scree, or rubble), and their corresponding factors are jettisoned. Keep in mind that logic and theory always trump a subjective visualization of the graph: the graph should never supplant sound theory.

If there are no clear factors, one may need to rerun the analysis with dropping problematic items (e.g., low-loadings, cross-loadings, or one item loading onto one factor). This must be done judiciously and without disregard to potentially bona fide neuropsychological constructs.

Rotating Factors

Although the premise for factor extraction is to determine the number of factors that comprise the test items, it remains a crude mathematical abstraction (DeVellis, 2003) that requires additional throughput for an intelligible solution. Rotation maximizes high loadings and minimizes low loadings to achieve simple structure. As DeVellis (2003) states, rotation achieves clarity by seeking factors that result in each items loading substantially on only one factor.

Factor rotation is used to position the factors to form coherent, conceptually identifiable constructs. Factor rotation improves the meaningfulness, dependability, and reproducibility of factors (Ford et al., 1986). There are two forms of rotation: orthogonal and oblique.

Orthogonal Rotation

In orthogonal rotation, the factors are considered independent or uncorrelated. Although this makes for a simpler solution than oblique rotation, it is often based on false pretenses. It is not uncommon for neuropsychological tests—even though they purportedly measure separate constructs—to be correlated. The final product is found by examining the factor loadings on the rotated factor matrix.

Oblique Rotation

In oblique rotation, independence of factors is disallowed, and the factors are able to correlate. Oblique rotation more accurately represents the complexity of the examined variables because constructs in the "real world" are rarely uncorrelated (Ford et al., 1986).

Theory should dictate which rotation method is used. The simplicity of orthogonal rotation methods is appealing, whereas, oblique rotations are often considered problematic because of the conceptual overlap among the factors (since they are allowed to be correlated and are not forced into independent factors). If oblique rotation is implemented, the researcher gleans his or her information (i.e., items loadings) from the pattern matrix.

Preliminary exploration of item correlations is acceptable. Some choose to begin with an oblique rotation, and if the resultant factor correlations are not high (as identified within the factor correlation matrix), an orthogonal rotation is performed because of its simplicity. However, Fabrigar et al. (1999), among others, believe that it is hard to justify *not* using an oblique rotation in EFA.

How Do I Name or Interpret the Factors?

A cogent factor analysis will result in high factor loadings without cross-loadings (i.e., high loadings one more than one dimension), plus several variables loading strongly on each factor. A cross-loading item—generally—is an item that loads at 0.32 or higher on two or more factors. A factor with fewer than three items is considered weak and unstable.

Examining the factor loadings of each item on each factor will help you determine: on which factor does an item correlate with the most, and the clinical relationship of the item to the other highly loaded items within one factor. Common rule is that any loading equal to or greater than 0.40 on a factor should be considered significant and used in helping to define the factor. Values below 0.32 are considered poor (Tabachnick & Fidell, 2001), as any such items share less than 10% of overlapping variance with the other items with that factor (Costello & Osborne, 2005).

There are several problems with EFA. As DeVellis (2003) cautions, "choosing a label for a factor…is not the same as establishing validity" (pg. 126). In other words, it is possible that findings are sample specific and reflect sample-specific variability rather than veritable neuropsychological constructs. However, there are ways of bolstering the theories derived from EFA. Although beyond the scope of this chapter, some of these methods include cross-validation (running either a confirmatory factor analysis or an additional EFA with the same items in a separate sample), or using monte-carlo simulations to substantiate the factor structure.

The Adventitious Extras of FA

Comparing Factor Scores

It is sometimes desired to compare groups on particular constructs. For example, one might like to compare two groups on different aspects of depression (affective, behavioral, and cognitive). One could administer a self-administered questionnaire like the Beck Depression Inventory (Beck, Ward, Mendelson, Mock, & Erbaugh, 1961), subject it to factor analysis, and yield orthogonal factors of depression (instead of simply comparing groups on the composite score). One can then compare (using t-tests or ANOVAs) the groups on each factor. This might be particularly useful, for example, if one group experienced significant behavioral effects related to an illness, rather than to depression. Therefore, examining groups only on the composite measure may dissemble veritable differences in depression between groups.

Using Factor Scores as a Step in Subsequent Analysis

*E*FA can be a preliminary step for regression analysis. As one fundamental assumption not to violate in regression analysis is multicollinearity—as predictor variables can share much conceptual overlap and cause problems for interpretation. EFA can be used to yield orthogonal factors. These factors, since they are now independent and conceptually unrelated, can then be used as predictors in a regression analysis.

Common Sense

Unlike similar factor-analytic designs that require statistical criteria and a priori methods, EFA relies on these rather subjective methods of inspection. However, nothing can replace common sense. Once you have examined the factors, it is important to look at the content of the items to determine whether they make theoretical sense. Does, for example, the items that were supposed to be assessing learning and memory load together, or are they split asunder with no apparent rhyme or reason?

In addition, peculiar loadings may represent sample specific findings. On the other hand, they may reveal something about the data that was not readily apparent. It may guide further inquiry into neuropsychological theory.

Simple Example of EFA in Neuropsychology

Although from fabricated data, the purpose of this simple example is purely illustrative. I have no intentions to expound complex mathematical or technical precepts. This example is based on an EFA from nine neuropsychological test scores. I have not included a scree plot, as they are generally self-explanatory.

As you can see from Table 4.2 (from an orthogonally rotated exploratory factor analysis) four factors were derived. The first step would be to examine either by row, or by column, the factor loadings. For example, starting down the first column (factor 1), there are three high factor loadings: immediate recall, delayed recall, and recognition. Based on the conceptual relationship among these tests, one might label this factor learning/memory. Perusing down the second column (factor 2), there are three tests with high loadings: SDMT, Grooved Pegboard Test, and Trail Making Test, Part A. What these tests share in common is motor and processing speed. Hence, one might decide to label this factor "speed." As for the third column (factor 3), there are two test scores with high loadings: Wisconsin Card Sorting Test and Trail Making Test, Part B. These tests are reminiscent of executive cognition: set-shifting and higher-order concept formation. One might therefore label this factor "executive functioning." Last, the Clock Drawing Test represents the fourth factor, and might be labeled spatial cognition. Of course, this is merely as an exemplar; no factor analysis should retain one item to represent an entire factor. This would be ill-judged and irreproducible and more than likely sample specific.

Of course, factor loadings do not generally slice and dice so evenly. And it is not uncommon to have items that load high on more than one factor. For example, in this example (seen in Table 4.2), Trail Making Test, Part B loads not only with the Wisconsin Card Sorting Test to represent executive functioning, but it also loads relatively well with the second factor (i.e., 0.48), which we have labeled "speed." Of course, this is not all that surprising given the Trail Making Test, Part B is a speeded test (the Wisconsin Card Sorting Test, however, is clearly not).

Table 4.2 Hypothetical factor structure of nine neuropsychological test scores (from a total of six tests)

	Factor 1	Factor 2	Factor 3	Factor 4
HVLT-R immediate recall	0.67	0.32	0.20	0.07
HVLT-R delayed recall	0.77	0.27	0.19	0.11
HVLT-R recognition	0.81	0.13	0.15	0.18
SDMT	0.15	0.88	0.22	0.31
Grooved pegboard test	0.13	0.65	0.19	0.27
Wisconsin card sorting test	0.07	0.04	0.91	0.25
Trail making test, Part A	0.18	0.56	0.23	0.21
Trail making test, Part B	0.14	0.48	0.79	0.24
Clock drawing test	0.09	0.11	0.35	0.86

Note: SDMT Symbol digit modalities test, *HVLT-R* Hopkins verbal learning test—Revised

Summary

EFA is a data reduction procedure that seeks to examine the variation and covariation among a large set of test scores. The tests/scores, which correlate highly, are considered to invoke similar cognitive processes. These items are clustered to form distinct cognitive functions, for example, attention, language, memory, executive function, and spatial cognition. EFA is a theory-building procedure that has helped to conceive neuropsychology as a discipline.

The purpose of this chapter was to purposefully exclude mathematical and mind-numbing precepts of EFA. Rather, a conceptual overview regarding EFA was provided. The role of EFA as a data reduction procedure emulates an important principle in psychological thought: parsimony. The role of EFA is appropriate for items and tests that are considered to measure separate—either uncorrelated (orthogonal) or correlated (oblique)—aspects of cognitive function. The steps in EFA were discussed as well, including selection of an appropriate model and extraction method (e.g., principal components analysis), selecting factors to retain, choosing appropriate rotation methods based on the relatedness among factor scores and test items, and characterizing the constructs which comprise a number of items. A few additional uses of EFA in research (e.g., to eliminate multicollinearity of predictors in a multiple regression analysis) were discussed, as well as a simple description of EFA to interpret a data set consisting of nine neuropsychological scores.

Chapter 5
Normative Data in Clinical Neuropsychology

Introduction

Clinical neuropsychology, like any other health profession, attempts to define the boundaries between normality and abnormality. Before we can identify, diagnose, intervene, or prognose, we must have criteria by which to classify whether or not a condition of interest is met. This lends itself to constructing seemingly arbitrary demarcations: a point at which we must call a score abnormal, and perhaps the ability responsible for such performance, impaired. This has its weaknesses in that it involves pigeonholing continuous phenomena into categories. However, this is the nature of clinical science. We must relinquish perhaps more accurate dimensional aspects of human experience and supplant them with more rigid and imprecise categories. Yet, done so judiciously yield, clinically relevant information.

Unfortunately, trying to render dichotomous decisions in the real world is not without problems, nor is it without heated debate. Nonetheless, it is not only easier to pin down and study phenomena when they are categorical, but we are also better able to provide more discrete and definitive conclusions to patients and their families. This scientifically driven process involves identifying a particular human experience, developing standardized criteria by which to sample and measure such experiences, and outlining the distributions of these characteristics among the population. This allows us to determine whether performance on neuropsychological testing is average (in comparison to a population) or abnormal (compared to an individual's premorbid functioning).

Providing objective criteria for determining impairment from normality helps bring structure and stability to clinical neuropsychology. It is when test performance hovers around these arbitrary cutoffs that we have most difficulty in our diagnostic certainty. It is here where we must decide among a relative weakness, a minor cognitive inefficiency, or the very earliest stages of an insidious and progressive illness.

D.A. Maroof, *Statistical Methods in Neuropsychology: Common Procedures Made Comprehensible*, DOI 10.1007/978-1-4614-3417-7_5,

Like any other type of nosology or classification system, the reasoning behind trying to describe and define what is and is not normal has utilitarian values. And despite the vitriolic debate that it engenders, its ultimate purposes are for the better. Classification helps us bring order to chaos, and helps define that which is ill-defined. Further, being able to detect people who fall outside the boundaries of normality allows us to raise red flags and step in to begin treatment. It also allows us to intervene, discern possible etiologies for someone's difficulties, and at times, shape the trajectory of a person's current treatment. As an example of the latter, based on a patient's performance on cognitive testing and their history, we might determine that the difficulties they are experiencing on neuropsychological testing are not suggestive of a neurodegenerative illness, but rather, are more than likely caused by a number of powerful, and perhaps intoxicating, medicines. The recommended "treatment" might involve suggesting the patient's medication regimen be re-examined to consider whether certain medicines should be reduced or eliminated.

All this would not be possible without systematic methods for examining neuropsychological functioning. However, as is evident in the last case, a thorough history is essential to supplement the data. Normative data allows us to standardize neuropsychological test scores so that we can gain an appreciation for performance on tests in the general population. We use these data to benchmark individual patient's performance. It is not only the severity of a deficit that provides clinically meaningful information, but the pattern of deficits as well as the context in which they are presented (e.g., depression). Clinical judgment should always supplement and at times trump decisions conferred by the data.

The purpose of this chapter is to discuss two general purposes of normative data as well as common approaches to constructing normative data; conventional norms, overlapping cell norms, regression-based norms, and robust norms. Each method's advantages and disadvantages are discussed.

General Categories for Normative Data

Normative data provide the distribution of performances in a specific sample on any given test. This pooled performance serves as the benchmark for evaluating individual performances on testing. For example, a person who earns a Full Scale IQ of 100 indicates that, in contrast with the population IQ, he performed better than 50% of those in the reference (population) group. However, this tells us nothing about *changes* in a patient's neuropsychological functioning (i.e., has his intellect been compromised?).

Busch, Chelune, and Suchy (2006) describe two very different purposes of normative data: descriptive and diagnostic. And, depending on the referral question and purpose of the neuropsychological examination (e.g., is this person mentally retarded; has this person shown a cognitive decline from his premorbid abilities?), a particular normative standard should be implemented and/or emphasized.

For normative data that are descriptive, the purpose of the evaluation is to determine how an individual is performing relative to the population. The question is, "where does this person stand in comparison to a particular reference population?" According to Busch et al. (2006), clinicians may, for example, use such information descriptively to illustrate patients' standings (e.g., within the low average or average range).

For diagnostic purposes, normative data are used to judge whether a patient's cognition is impaired or not. More specifically, the clinician seeks to determine whether a patient's cognitive functioning represents a change (e.g., decline) from his putative premorbid abilities. In this case, the individual's performance is compared to his estimated premorbid status (e.g., via word reading measures, and/or educational or occupational attainment).

As Busch et al. (2006) further explain, the differences between descriptive and diagnostic norms are fundamentally different both conceptually and psychometrically. For descriptive purposes, the construct (e.g., memory) measured is assumed to be normally distributed. Conclusions regarding this type of normative standard can thus be established from a Gaussian distribution. This means, information regarding standard scores and percentiles can be easily computed based on mathematical "givens" for normally distributed data.

At the other end of the spectrum, though often used in conjunction with population-based norming, diagnostic use of normative data centers around an illness-based approach. Essentially, these constructs do not assume a normal distribution. This is because they are highly skewed (i.e., negatively skewed, since "normals" performances are generally errorless or are nearly errorless) and have minimal dispersion in scores. Language problems, orientation, a homonymous hemianopsia, and so on, are relevant to this type of norming procedure. For example, it makes no sense to describe a patient's orientation as within the average range (as tests are for descriptive purposes). Instead, a person's orientation could either be normal (intact) or abnormal. Similarly, in a patient who displays a Broca's aphasia (nonfluent aphasia), the clinician does not dither over whether the aphasia is in the "average" range. Rather, a Broca's aphasia is by definition pathognomonic and considered—no matter how severe—abnormal.

Using Normative Data in Clinical Neuropsychology

Blindly using any available normative data is unprofessional and unethical. We have to examine the makeup of the normative sample—are they similar in age and education for example—before we compare our patient with the norm. In addition, there are several assumptions that we hold when calculating certain standard scores. For example, when calculating a z-score, we assume that the scores are from a normal distribution. This is not the case for many neuropsychological tests. There are ways of dealing with this, including using cumulative frequency distributions for determining the ranking of a patient's test performance. We are aware, through common knowledge and empirical validation, that several factors can influence how one performs on a particular test. So, things like age, education, sex, and even race, need to be taken into account when determining whether one's performance on a task is "normal." It gets tricky. Not every test is affected the same.

None of us are the same, especially when it comes to how we perform on neurocognitive testing. We would expect the performance on a memory test between an 18-year-old and an 80-year-old, holding all other relevant factors constant (e.g., education, sex, etc.), to differ. We would expect that an 18-year-old would (and should) outperform someone 62 years his or her senior. Why? Because neuropsychologists have their own "internal" norms for how we would expect certain persons to perform on neuropsychological tests. However, in order to add some objectivity to this process, we have normative data (e.g., means and standard deviations) of test scores, which are derived from small to large samples of persons free of any neurological or psychiatric illness, or any type of historical information (e.g., history of head trauma) that might contribute to poorer performance on baseline cognitive testing. The measures of central tendency and dispersion from this normal population are used as benchmarks for which we can compare patients' performance. This way, we can determine whether a patient's score—from which we infer performance or the integrity of a cognitive ability—is what might be expected given his or her demographic constitution or whether both the extent and severity of cognitive function indicate the presence of a malignant neurological condition.

Importance of Choosing the "Right" Normative Data

There is no perfect normative data set to use, rather, there are usually more appropriate normative data sets to use. Selecting the most appropriate normative data for your patient is just as important as the validity of a test. In other words, even if your measure has shown adequate construct validity, the fact that you are administering the same test to someone who is well outside the normative sample (for example, using normative data from persons over 80 years of age to examine memory performance in a 35-year old) reveals nothing. After all, we use normative data to determine whether patients' scores are low or high relative to the population, as well as whether they represent changes from the patient's estimated premorbid abilities. Next, we determine whether these low or high scores reflect inefficiencies, deficiencies, or impairments in performance and functioning. Clearly, this has tremendous implications for diagnosis, recommendations, and ultimate treatment of the patient.

Several different methods have been used to derive normative data. Generally, normative data can fall into one of two categories: discrete or continuous norms (Parmenter, 2010). Discrete norms (including stratified norms using overlapping cell means), as well as regression-based techniques and robust norming will be discussed.

Discrete (Stratified) Norms

In discrete norms, which we are most familiar with, we are usually presented with nonoverlapping successive age bands (e.g., 20–29 years old, 30–39 years old, etc.), perhaps stratified further by education. Means and standard deviations within each age band are provided. Raw scores from patients can be used to calculate z-scores (standard scores), and hence, the relative standing of that score can be obtained.

The process of scoring a patient's performance is quite simple. For most situations (e.g., if the data from the normative sample are normally distributed) we take each raw score (e.g., how many words the person was able to recall on a list-learning measure), and calculate a standard score (i.e., z-score) to determine 1—*direction*: are they at, above, or below the mean, and 2—*extent*: how far that person is from the mean (e.g., one standard deviation below the mean). Converting all of the persons raw test scores into standard scores allows us to compare apples and oranges. That is, we can compare the differences among all other tests (e.g., memory, processing speed, etc.). Examining the pattern of test performance often allows us to both diagnose (e.g., dementia) and infer pathology (e.g., Alzheimer disease).

Parementer et al. (2010) note that a main limitation of discrete norms is that an individual's raw score might yield very dissimilar standings (e.g., percentiles) if the person is on the cusp of a different age band. For example, if someone is tested a day prior to his or her birthday, a particular score might fall within the borderline range. However, had this individual been tested one day later. this same score might have fallen in the low average to average range.

The ambiguity of precise values in discrete norms' age bands is a major concern. For example, the means within each age band is an unknown, and although a patient who is 51 years old seems appropriate for an age band 50–59, it may be that the normative sample that makes up this age band has a mean age of 58. On the other hand, the age band preceding (i.e., 40–49) has a mean age of 49. Thus, the lower age band is technically more appropriate for this patient. However, this information is diluted when using discrete norms. As Busch et al. (2006) also mention, the data within each age band may not be normally distributed, making the interpretations based on the psychometric properties of a Gaussian distribution (i.e., the percentage of persons who fall within certain standard deviations from the mean) inappropriate.

Overlapping Cell Norms

Overlapping cell norms help to make better use of all-too-often limited normative tests data (Pauker, 1988). In this procedure, overlapping cell norms are created at specified age midpoints. Thus, participants appear in one or more of the adjacent cells, but the cells that are juxtaposed with one another differ in their midpoint means, but overlap in range. The advantage of this approach over stratified norms is that the group means are more stable, resulting in less abrupt shifts in means between age blocks. Another advantage is that it requires far fewer participants than other methods of normative creation (since the same participants are used repeatedly).

Regression-Based Norms

Regression-based norms differ in that they help capture and control for more specific individual characteristics when examining a person's neuropsychological test performance. Most neuropsychological test performances are affected by age and education. Ethnicity and sex play a role in tests as well. The utility of regression-based norms is instead of using crude demographic bands to calculate standard scores, an individual's performance is tailored to his or her unique attributes—age, education, and sex, for example. These demographic variables are used in a multiple regression analysis. Equations derived from a multiple regression analysis are used to predict test performance based on a patient's demographic characteristic, making normative conversions highly individualized (Testa, Winicki, Pearlson, Gordon, & Schretlen, 2009). As these authors further note, the discrepancy between a person's predicted and actual scores is evaluated against a distribution of discrepancy scores shown by a normative sample. Large discrepancies (e.g., a predicted score for a memory test is higher than the persons' obtained score) suggest a decline in function.

One of the advantages of regression-based norms has to do with avoiding the prohibitive sample sizes that are required if one wants to use conventional norms that stratify for several demographic variables, drastically diminishing the sample size of each cell.

Robust Norms

The crux of robust norming (Sliwinski, Lipton, Buschke, & Stewart, 1996) is to refine the true meaning of normative data. In essence, normative data should reflect how persons who are free of any disease process perform on cognitive testing.

Robust norms attempt to circumvent the problems typically associated with cross-sectional methods for obtaining normative data by compiling and calculating norms prospectively. In this manner, participants included in the normal data collection who develop a cognitive disorder (e.g., Alzheimer disease) "down the road" are removed from the final normative sample. This way, the final normative sample is a more accurate reflection of "normal" persons' performance.

As Holtzer, Goldin, Zimmerman, Katz, Buschke, and Lipton (2008) point out, excluding individuals who develop dementia at some point following their baseline assessment will reduce the variability in normative data (since the range of scores will not be as great since persons who likely scored quite low at baseline are excluded), and increase the mean values (excluding those in the lower end of the normal range will result in high scores altogether, which will increase the mean value). This will yield a more reliable estimate of normal cognition that is likely to detect the very earliest stages of dementia syndromes.

Another strength of developing robust norms is being able to deal with attrition (Holtzer et al., 2008). In other words, persons who do not return for follow-up assessment might differ in fundamental ways from those who do return. Those who do not return for follow-up assessment might be more cognitively impaired, more physically limited, have lower socioeconomic status (e.g., perhaps they were unable to afford transportation), live in certain areas with transportation that is not as efficient and more challenging. So, including individuals in cross-sectional norms who would have otherwise been lost to follow-up may also wreak havoc on the variability of test scores, decrease means, and be less sensitive to cognitive decline, making those in the very earliest stages of disease more difficult to detect.

Summary

This chapter discussed general principles of normative data, including describing the fundamental difference between descriptive and diagnostic norming. Further, brief descriptions of norming procedures were provided, including that of discrete norms, overlapping cell norms, regression-based norms, and robust norms, as well as some of their advantages and disadvantages.

Chapter 6
Covariates and Covariance Analyses

Introduction

A confounding variable is the bane of every clinician's and researcher's existence. A confounding variable is anything that can affect (or effect) an outcome measure, principally performance on neuropsychological testing, and is not of primary relevance in clinical practice or experimentation. However, their presence interferes with the ability to descry particular phenomenon, and either clouds or deceives neuropsychologists' judgments by distorting the relationships among variables.

Depression, motivation (or lack thereof), fatigue, age, and even the time of day, can serve to "hoodwink" both the tests and the clinician. Such factors can bring unnecessary "noise" to neuropsychological test performance. However, knowledge and appraisal of relevant factors that might confound test performance and clinical judgment at least provides some modicum of control of these possible influences, and therefore makes possible for more refined, precise results and decisions. Nonetheless, such variables make interpretation and clinical judgment challenging, as they can mislead and misinform both test results and the ensuing inferences.

Because nothing exists in a vacuum in either clinical practice or research, we must continually evaluate, and frequently measure, these variables. In practice and research we use both clinical interview and neuropsychological tests. A comprehensive understanding of the patient provides an avenue to detect and diminish the relevance of factors that appear to be inconsequential.

On interview, a clinician elicits information about a person's schooling: did they experience any trouble in acquiring fundamental skills in reading, writing, or arithmetic? Any such troubles may suggest a developmental or learning disorder, and these vulnerabilities can affect current test performance and interpretation. A patient's mood, prior neuropsychological testing, as well as his comprehensive medical and psychiatric history should be culled. It behooves the clinician to determine whether

D.A. Maroof, *Statistical Methods in Neuropsychology: Common Procedures Made Comprehensible*, DOI 10.1007/978-1-4614-3417-7_6,

anything in a person's history might represent a possible impediment to test performance, and hence, clinical inferences. The clinician has to decide whether some variables are merely superfluous and "road-side attractions" and more likely to represent red herrings.

Research is equally difficult, except that it is a group, nomothetic method, rather than an individual, idiographic approach. However, research allows for more quantifiable and precise measurement of the influence of particular confounding variables. Together, clinical experience and research provide fodder for each other: clinical hunches and tentative hypotheses can be examined in experimental paradigms, and significant findings from research studies can inform clinical practice.

Purposes of This Chapter

The purposes of this chapter are to provide a general overview of how covariates can be managed in clinical practice, and restrained in neuropsychological research. As for the latter, this includes how covariates may be detected for inclusion in statistical analysis, and some of the pitfalls and myths of covariates. Indiscriminate use of covariates in research is cautioned, but when used properly and judiciously, covariates can help provide a clearer understanding of the relationships among variables of interest.

Common statistical approaches that allow for the control of covariates, namely analysis of covariance (ANCOVA) and multiple regression will be discussed. However, there are a plethora of statistical models that allow for covariates (e.g., multivariate analysis of covariance; MANCOVA: an extension of MANOVA). Simple examples using neuropsychological data will be provided to help elucidate the use and interpretation of covariance analysis

Confounding Variables in Clinical Practice

In clinical practice, we are often faced with the daunting task of traversing persons' life histories to explain why they are performing at a certain level on neuropsychological testing. We may have a patient that presents with psychiatric illness, a history of a brain injury, and/or a family history of Alzheimer's disease. We must wade through the patient's current and past events, trait and state variables, family history, and all the other nooks and crannies. Notwithstanding these factors, we are often relied upon or perhaps delegated the task of, determining whether a person's performance on neuropsychological testing can be attributed to one underlying process—yet, because of the scad of potential etiologies, we must decide whether a number of "patient" variables are significant or inconsequential to a patient's current complaints. If we are unsure, we espouse a "wait and see" approach, or seek which factors can be controlled and/or modified—vitamin deficiencies, the number and type of medicines a patient is taking. If clinically significant changes (e.g., improved cognitive function) occur following modifications to a patient's "life-style," we can be sure that other potentially irreversible etiologies that were looming large can now fall by the wayside.

Clinicians warranted. It is in everyone's (clinician and patient) best interest to assess all potentially relevant factors in explaining a patient's neuropsychological problems. Slapdash assessments and inconclusive diagnoses do a disservice to the patient, and are likely to leave the referral source feeling empty handed and ill-equipped to further care for the patient.

We want to avoid or at least mitigate such ill-conceived conclusions both in clinical practice and research. One way of doing so is through comprehensive evaluations. In clinical practice, this allows for sound conceptualization, and in research, an unambiguously lucid relationship between an independent and a dependent variable. Being thorough one can gain greater confidence and conviction in test results and clinical decisions.

Several variables we encounter are likely to affect cognition in some way or another. We know this based on both clinical lore and empirical investigations. We must weigh vascular risk factors and vascular disease, family history of suspected or confirmed neurologic illness, and the unsubstantiated and possibly erroneous self-report of past head injuries and their severity. However, what these variables all have in common is that they are considered confounding, or nuisance variables: a patient's experiences and current life conditions that may befuddle the clinical picture and make it difficult and sometimes impossible to proffer a parsimonious, and unambiguous diagnosis.

Confounding variables vie for attention, and the clinician must decide which of the numerous variables are the most cogent and conspicuous so as to be considered a "cause" (or part-cause) of the patient's cognitive and emotional difficulties on neuropsychological examination.

Confounding Variables in Research

A confounding or nuisance variable in research is any variable that varies systematically with the dependent variable under study. Age and education, for example, are commonly associated with neuropsychological test performance. Those who have advanced degrees are more likely to outperform those who only completed the fifth grade. Therefore, if the question is whether men and women differ on a cognitive test, we must first ensure that they not differ significantly on a host of potentially important confounding variables. If there exists such a difference, inclusion of one or more variables in the statistical model may be necessary to curb their influence over primary outcome measures. This allows the researcher to examine the specific relationship between independent (e.g., sex) and dependent (e.g., cognition) variables without any interference from confounding variables.

As we have come to learn, confounding or nuisance variables are aptly named because they can leave us terribly nonplussed and irritated, mainly because they make our job of dismantling group differences all the more difficult. When we attempt to rein in on such confounding variables in research, they are referred to as covariates. In other words, confounding variables are termed covariates when we use statistical corrections to attenuate their influence on our outcome measure. We may determine that differences in age, education, or intelligence among groups are too great so as not to go uncorrected. Using these variables as covariates in statistical analysis allows us to diminish their affects on the primary outcome variable, allowing for a more "diaphanous" look at the dependent variable.

As I mentioned, covariates are variables that "covary" or change systematically as a function of the dependent variable. In statistical analyses, we are in fact stripping the confounding variables effect from the dependent variable, providing a purer, and at times, more sensitive look at the differences between the independent variables.

Without control of confounding variables, via covariance analysis, the independent variable's effect on the dependent variable (s), or merely the relationship between the two, is often muddled. By using covariates in research, and by achieving reasonable methodological control of third variable and extraneous influences, we feel secure in asserting that our findings are strongly associated, and perhaps the result of, a specific factor (e.g., brain injury, neurodegenerative illness, psychiatric illness, etc.), rather than to disparities from other plausible influences.

Without attention to and an understanding of confounding variables in research, variables that were overlooked in the design and analysis, render the results, and our conclusions, specious. The reason being is simple: if variables that vary systematically with an outcome variable are not tended to, they may explain a significant amount of the variance in the dependent variable, clouding the independent contribution of the independent variable. For example, comparing neuropsychological functioning in patients with left and right strokes may be baseless if those with right and left hemisphere lesions differ on noteworthy characteristics: age, education, intelligence, sex, etc.

Main Goal of Using Covariates

The overarching purpose of using covariates in statistical analyses is to increase the signal to noise ratio. The goal is to determine the individual influence) between independent variables by having other potentially relevant and plausibly shroud veritable mean differences.

Covariates are a very important part of research design and statistical analysis. They allow us to control for extraneous and adventitious factors that may be nearly impossible to isolate and/or manipulate in real life. Generally speaking there are two ways of controlling for confounding variables: methodologically and statistically. Methodologically is a "built-in" approach wherein the study design prevents certain factors, whereas the statistical approach involves mathematical corrections of the covariates' influence (of course, after the data have been collected).

Methodological Control of Confounding Variables

Methodological refers to the *method or design* by which the participants are randomly selected and assigned. It also refers to the procedures employed and the tests administered. Both are critically important to achieve control of extraneous factors (i.e., confounding/nuisance variables).

Methods and Procedures

Any worthy research paper, under the participants section, will include a fairly lengthy list of exclusionary criteria for persons in the study: a history of a traumatic brain injury, alcohol dependence, psychiatric illness, certain medicines, or developmental or neurological problems that are likely to affect cognitive test performance. This is a way of methodological control. It is essential to exclude participants who have conditions likely to affect—or vary systematically with the dependent variable—neuropsychological performance. By eliminating particular participants, the resultant sample is more homogeneous. Winnowing down the range of possible confounding variables removes possible sources of officious noise.

This is the foremost goal of an experiment, to have the most confidence that the dependent (outcome measure) is *dependent* on the influence of the independent variable. That memory performance is dependent on the sex of the participants, rather than on a history of neurological illness, drug use, or neurodevelopmental disorder, is critical for preventing our results from not being obscured by peripheral, yet perhaps equally important influences. Unfortunately, we sacrifice external validity—the extent to which we can generalize the results of our finding to the "real world"—for internal validity (the extent to which our results are bona fide and accurate reflections of what is measured). This is because in the real world, meaning clinical practice, it is uncommon to encounter persons without medical or psychiatric or other life circumstances that can affect their neuropsychological test performance. It is a rarity to come across persons without remarkable life events.

Methodological control often occurs during participant selection; it is a process approach. However, there are ways of using methodological control by stratifying the sample and running separate analyses. For example, instead of using sex as a covariate in analysis, if there are a large number of available participants, analysis of only males or females, or only those in a certain age or education bracket should be considered. This way, the results cannot be attributed to sex, age, or education. This is not very common, however, as such analyses requires a large number of participants.

Tests Administered

Tests to Exclude Participants

The neuropsychological tests administered can be used, either in isolation or in combination, to form groups of participants so as to gain control of certain variables. For example, participants who score below a certain value on the Mini Mental State Exam are often excluded from analysis so as not to have persons who might be demented to be included and influence the overall results. Similarly, persons who score above a certain criterion on a depression inventory might be disregarded so as not to include persons whose depression could account for a good amount of the variance in the dependent variable.

Tests to Include and Group Participants

Performance on tests can be used not merely to exclude participants, but to categorize and allocate them into particular groups. For example, a researcher interested in examining certain cognitive abilities in gifted individuals (i.e., IQ greater than 130) would need to first determine whether participants are in fact "gifted." Ergo, participants will be included based on test performance.

This process is similar to examining differences among patients: persons with and without a disease, with and without diabetes, or with and without anxiety, for example. Their status alone dictates the group to which they belong.

Test Scores Used Directly in Statistical Analyses

Tests are important because they attach value to hypothetical constructs like attention, memory, language, and executive cognition. These values—the scores and ratings from measures—can be used in statistical analysis. So, instead of using scores on neuropsychological tests to separate or exclude participants, we can incorporate test scores directly into the analysis so as to statistically correct for their influence on measures of primary relevance. The advantage of this procedure is that we can see how the covariate is related to the dependent variable and we do not lose participants merely because of their scores or performances on certain measures. For example, including age, education, scores on inventories of mood, etc. can be integrated with analysis. The scores will adjust the dependent variables based on the relationships between the covariates and the outcome measures.

Researchers often incorporate covariates, often because it has been done in most other similar studies. Of course, we are studying brain–behavior relationships, so unless you are studying persons with Parkinson's disease, any participant with Parkinson's disease is likely to be excluded from your study.

Statistical Control of Confounding Variables

Methodological control often involves the intentional omission of certain variables, whereas statistical control involves explicitly incorporating the confounding variables into the statistical models. As an example of the former, when participants are being considered for inclusion of a study, many are purposefully excluded because of certain characteristics that can render the interpretations of a study difficult. Statistical control is a solution to the inevitability of sample characteristics that could not have been managed or factored out of the design. Groups may differ on age, education, intelligence, depression—many variables, unless matched for, will often be problematic if not partialed out of the analysis.

There are two commonly used statistical methods for adjusting for covariates: mean difference analyses (e.g., Analysis of Covariance; ANCOVA) and regression-based procedures (e.g., multiple regression). ANCOVA will be discussed in some detail. Since multiple regression is already covered elsewhere in this book, it is only briefly discussed.

Analysis of Covariance

ANCOVA examines whether mean differences on an *adjusted* dependent/outcome variable are due to chance. So, it is an extension of ANOVA, since ANOVA examines whether mean differences on an unadjusted (original metric) variable differs between groups. The difference between ANCOVA and ANOVA lies in examining whether comparison of groups involves *adjusted* (*ANCOVA*) rather than unadjusted (without adjustment) (ANOVA) means. In other words, the effects of one or more covariate are partialed out or removed from the dependent variable. This way, ANCOVA provides a clearer picture of group differences on the outcome primary variable (Fig. 6.1).

As an example, if one were to examine sex differences on memory performance, covariates might include certain hormone levels, age, and education. Bear in mind that if groups do not differ on variables, they are not included as covariates (e.g., if men and women are found to differ in age based on a t-test). It is only when groups differ on plausibly salient variables that they serve as covariates. This way, we can achieve greater confidence that any differences between the two groups are due to the independent variable, and are not being influenced by the covariates that are equally likely to explain a good portion of the variance in the dependent variable.

Three Main Reasons for Choosing ANCOVA

1. To reduce the error term: the covariance between the covariate and the dependent variable allows us to remove systematic variance from the error term.

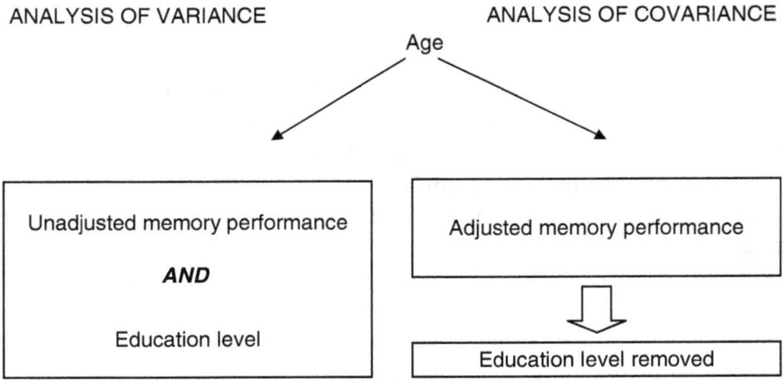

Fig. 6.1 Difference between analysis of variance (ANOVA) and analysis of covariance (ANCOVA) wherein the effects of the covariate are partialed out of the dependent variable; the main focus in ANOVA and ANCOVA is unadjusted and adjusted means, respectively

2. Nonexperimental designs: to adjust posttest scores based on pretest scores.
3. Follow-up analyses (i.e., after a significant multivariate analysis of variance; MANOVA), referred to as stepdown analysis.

Reducing the Error Term

In experimental designs, where participants are randomly selected and randomly assigned, ANCOVA helps remove any systematic variance from the error term. This is considered the most appropriate use for ANCOVA, as it is within the context of a true experimental design, and any variables (e.g., test scores) that might covary with the outcome variable of interest are considered for inclusion in the analysis as a covariate. The purpose of ANCOVA is therefore to improve the sensitivity of the test so that a purer relationship between the independent variable and the dependent variable can be assessed. The main advantage of an experimental design is that one can infer causality.

NonExperimental Designs

In this case, ANCOVA is used as a matching procedure, wherein group differences are compared after adjusting the dependent variable on one or more potentially threatening covariates.

For example, suppose patients with bipolar affective illness and unipolar depression were to be compared on neuropsychological tests. Of course, this is by definition a nonexperimental design because the illness *defines* the groups and decides in which group they lay. These are referred to as quasi-independent variables (and hence, a quasi-experimental design—one cannot randomly assign persons who have already been assigned by their diagnosis). Once the participants are selected for inclusion in the study, they will be compared on a number of variables: age, distribution of sex, education, intelligence, etc.

If the study were examining verbal fluency, for example, and the two groups significantly differed on any potentially relevant confound, the variable(s) might be considered as a covariate so that differences between groups could be examined as if things were "equal." If, for example, the two groups differed in education, using education as a covariate will compare those with bipolar affective illness and unipolar depression on verbal fluency *as if* they were equally educated.

Follow-Up Analyses

Following a significant omnibus MANOVA (with multiple dependent variables), a series of ANCOVAs, referred to as stepdown analysis, is an ideal post hoc technique. The procedure examines mean differences between groups on each dependent variable while covarying for all other dependent variables that were in the original analysis.

Specifically, the highest priority outcome variable is first examined in a univariate ANOVA. Then, the remaining outcome variables are tested in a series of ANCOVAs, with each successive variable tested with high-priority outcome variables as covariates to distinguish what, if anything, augments the results beyond the combination of outcome variables already tested.

As an example, suppose we were to compare patients with Alzheimer's disease (AD) and healthy elderly controls on cognitive tests. After a significant MANOVA (which included a number of cognitive tests), we assign the delayed recall score the highest priority since it represents the most common presenting symptom for patients with early AD. Next, we might want to add semantic fluency in an ANCOVA, using delayed recall as a covariate. The purpose would be to determine whether additional tests contribute to the results.

What to Look for in a Covariate: It's Not You, It's Me

Harlow (2005) delineated four characteristics to look for in determining the importance and proper use of a covariate.

First, the covariates should be at least moderately correlated with the dependent variable. According to Harlow, this means that the correlations should exceed a pearson's r of 0.3 (e.g., over 9% of the variance). Very little variance will be partialed out of the outcome variable before examining group differences. It is important to remember that for each additional covariate, the degrees of freedom for the error term is reduced, thereby attenuating the test statistic (for the ANCOVA) and making it more difficult to find a statistical significance.

Second, the covariates should be reliably measured: meaning a correlation greater than 0.70. This can be examined rather quickly by Cronbach's alpha for continuous variables.

Third, there should be low correlations among the covariates. If there are two or more covariates, and they are correlated, this leads to collinearity problems, yielding imprecise results.

Fourth, there should not be any appreciable correlation between the covariates and the independent variables in the model.

Assumptions of ANCOVA

Assumptions of ANCOVA are similar to most other univariate tests, and involve normality, linearity, homogeneity of variance, and reliability of covariates. These assumptions were covered earlier. However, there is one additional assumption specific to ANCOVA, referred to as homogeneity of regression slopes.

Homogeneity of Regression Slopes

Simply, this assumes that the relationship between the dependent variable and the covariate does not change as a function of the level of the independent variable. An interaction between the covariate and the independent variable indicates a violation of this assumption. This means that there is a different relationship between the covariate and the dependent variable at different levels of the independent variable.

Example of ANCOVA

As a simple example, supposed we were interested in examining mean differences between persons with multiple sclerosis and healthy elderly controls on a test of prospective memory. Prospective memory is essentially remembering to perform a planned action at a specific time. For example, recalling that at 3 PM an item has to be removed from the freezer to defrost for dinner is exhibiting intact prospective memory.

After recruiting participants and collecting data, we come to find out that the two groups differ in intelligence. After running a correlation between intelligence and prospective memory, it is determined that because those with lower intelligence perform more poorly on the prospective memory test, it might serve as a useful

Table 6.1 Abridged output of an ANCOVA comparing persons with multiple sclerosis and healthy controls on a test of prospective memory (PROMEM), using IQ as a covariate

Source	Mean square	F	Significance
Corrected model	189.25	72.5	0.02
Intercept	19.63	1.10	0.87
IQ	142.31	4.21	0.07
PROMEM	**188.55**	**5.98**	**0.03**
Error	12.72		
Total			

covariate in an ANCOVA. This means that, if both groups were equally smart, we want to determine whether there still exists a difference in prospective memory.

As seen in Table 6.1, intelligence was entered as a covariate in the ANCOVA. And, in the row labeled PROMEM, the results indicate that there is a significant difference between the groups even after equating them on intelligence.

Follow-Up Analysis of ANCOVA

I would be remiss if I did not mention follow-up analyses for statistical ANCOVAs. These are required when a significant omnibus ANCOVA involves more than two groups. In this case, it is still unclear as to where the significance lies: between groups 1 and 2, 1 and 3, or 2 and 3, for example.

Follow-up analysis for ANCOVA is very simple, and involves pairwise comparisons on the adjusted means.

Multiple Regression

Multiple regression is discussed in this book, so it will not be described in detail. However, its relevance for this chapter has to do with the use of covariates that are commonly included in analysis, including standard, stepwise, and/or hierarchical regression.

Briefly, this analysis allows us to predict a continuous dependent (criterion) variable from two or more independent (predictor) variables. For example, we might want to predict someone's performance on a test of memory from scores of processing speed, depression, and executive cognition. Let's say that we are interested in whether these variables predict memory performance above and beyond age and education. A hierarchical regression analysis could be used in which age and education are entered into Block 1, and neuropsychological variables in Block 2. If the neuropsychological variables remain significant in the second block, they clearly explain the variance in the dependent variable above and beyond that which is accounted for by age and education.

Misunderstandings and Misuses of Covariates

Despite the semblance of ANCOVA's versatility for experimental and nonexperimental designs, it is not uncommon for this procedure to be applied erroneously (Porter & Raudenbaush, 1987). Like any other statistical procedure, it should not be used as a blanket method for any type of design and any type of variable. Selection and use of covariates must be done so judiciously.

A major misconception in ANCOVA is a lack of theoretical and practical wherewithal on the part of the clinician/researcher. For example, if reading comprehension were compared among third, fourth, and fifth graders, it would be imprudent to control for age, as this variable is likely inextricably attached to grade level. It is an inherent attribute of grade. It would not make sense to say, "how would these elementary school in different grades perform on a test of reading comprehension if they were of similar age?" However, they are not of similar age mainly because they are in different grades!

Summary

This chapter discussed covariates and covariance analyses. First, a definition of a covariate or nuisance variable was provided, after which methods of control of covariates was partitioned into methodological and statistical control. Second, ANCOVA as a method for examining adjusted mean difference between groups (after having partialed out the effects of one or more covariates from the outcome/dependent variable) was discussed. Third, multiple regression analysis, another statistical model that allows for covariates, was briefly reviewed. Fourth, an example of how covariance analysis is used in neuropsychology was discussed to provided a clearer picture of how and why such methods might be appropriate or desirable in research. Last, brief misconceptions about ANCOVA were discussed.

Chapter 7
Regression Analyses

Introduction

Regression analyses are among the most commonly used statistical procedures in the social sciences. The reason for this is likely related to two fundamental goals of science: prediction and explanation of phenomena (Licht, 2001). With regression analyses, the goal is to predict or classify one variable—be it continuous (e.g., linear regression) or discrete (e.g., logistic regression) from one or more predictor or independent variables. Recall that prediction should be used appropriately to describe statistical analysis (in this case, regression) in which variables were measured systematically at separate time points: the predictor variable precedes the outcome/criterion variable. The term classification should be used when all variables (both predictors and criterion) are collected at roughly similar time points, with no methodological consideration for a temporal relationship. For this chapter, I use the terms interchangeably merely for stylistic variety.

Regression analysis examines the association between predictor and criterion variables. Exploring whether sex classifies performance on a test of executive cognition is an appropriate question for a regression analysis. The outcome or criterion variable, executive cognition, is regressed on the predictor variable, sex (male/female). As I will soon discuss, the criterion variable need not be continuous. In other words, one could reverse the above hypothesis and examine whether performance on a test of executive cognition (now the predictor variable) can classify whether a person is male or female (the dichotomous criterion variable). This would be appropriate for other kinds of regression analyses (e.g., logistic regression or discriminant function analysis). Regression analyses are also able to account for nonlinear relationships between the independent and dependent variables, such as curvilinear relationships.

Like most statistical procedures, regression serves many aims. It can be used as a method of covariate analysis (e.g., sequential regression, to be discussed shortly) to compare varying sets of predictor variables on an outcome measure (e.g., examining which memory test is best related to an ecologically valid marker), and perhaps

D.A. Maroof, *Statistical Methods in Neuropsychology: Common Procedures Made Comprehensible*, DOI 10.1007/978-1-4614-3417-7_7,

to generate a regression equation, which will allow the most important predictor variables to be established. This regression equation can then be used for future prediction. This process involves confirming an empirical relationship among variables in a study, and then applying these test statistics (i.e., the regression formula) at an individual level. This is the crux of clinical neuropsychological practice, particularly in evaluating premorbid intellect.

The Wechsler Test of Adult Reading (WTAR) (The Psychological Corporation, 2001) provides estimates of premorbid intellectual function based on regression equations that include demographics, a person's reading ability, or a combination of the two. Similarly, the Oklahoma Premorbid Intelligence Estimate (OPIE-3) (Schoenberg, Duff, Scott, Patton, & Adams, 2006) combines subtest raw scores from the WAIS-III (vocabulary, information, matrix reasoning, and picture completion) and demographic information (i.e., age, education, sex, ethnicity, and geographic region) to predict Full Scale IQ. Regression formulae are mathematical algorithms in which raw scores from an individual can be plugged. Premorbid intellectual functioning is the crux of neuropsychology as a primary target in clinical neuropsychology is to determine whether a person's cognitive function represents a decline from his premorbid abilities. Of course, we generally do not have baseline assessments of most persons to directly calculate a change in cognitive test performance, as suspected illness is generally the impetus for an evaluation (people do not undergo neuropsychological examinations like they do routine medical check-ups).

Regression is a correlational procedure; the intention of the researcher determines whether correlation analysis (e.g., bivariate or partial correlation) or a regression analysis is used. However, since regression analysis is mathematically a correlational procedure, only logic and experimental design establish whether cause can be inferred, and thus, truly declare prediction. Indiscriminately running a regression analysis and proclaiming a cause and effect relationship among variables is mere bunkum if predictor variables are culled well before the onset and measurement of an outcome measure—and with sufficient experimental control—then prediction is a propos. Otherwise, the researcher is mislabeling and misrepresenting the analysis.

Among the variables included in a regression analysis, theory, previous research findings, and at times, theory development (e.g., stepwise regression, to be discussed shortly) can provide direction. As a rule, regression will be most useful if the predictor variables are not highly correlated with one another but if each predictor variable is highly associated with the outcome or criterion variable. This makes sense as it signifies that each predictor variable contributes something unique to its prediction of the outcome, and thus, it yields a more thorough understanding of the phenomena under investigation.

As Tabachnick and Fidell (2001) highlight, both manipulative and non-manipulative variables should be considered for inclusion as predictor variables. In a regression analysis, a manipulative variable might be smoking and/or drinking habits, amount of exercise, or perhaps mood, whereas non-manipulative variables might include sex, genetics, and height. Whereas non-manipulative variables are by definition immutable, manipulative variables are modifiable, and this makes for clinically relevant information. That is, if the manipulative variables explain a large portion of the variance in the outcome measure treatment/intervention might be specifically geared toward those variables that can sway the outcome. For example, if depression explains work productivity to a large degree, rather than intelligence (which may be rather uncompromising to outside influences), then improvement of mood might be an effective and plausibly useful treatment recommendation.

There are several variations of these regression analyses, two of which will be discussed in this chapter: linear and curvilinear. The advantage of regression analyses over tests such as ANOVAs and MANOVAs is that we can earn a greater appreciation of the relationships among independent and dependent variables. This is because we can include continuous variables on either side of the equation. In ANOVAs and MANOVAs, we must categorize grouping (independent) variables, and simply compare mean differences among groups. The advantage of regression analyses is that predictor variables (independent variables) can be continuous (e.g., score on the Beck Depression Inventory) or categorical (e.g., whether or not the person has a history of a traumatic brain injury).

Simple (one independent variable) and multiple (i.e., several independent variables) analyses in regression are both considered univariate procedures. In fact, multiple regression analyses are referred to as multivariable rather than multivariate (Licht, 2001) methods. The term multivariate analysis is reserved for procedures in which there is more than one dependent variable, such as in multivariate analysis of variance (MANOVA). Regression analyses, as discussed in this chapter, include only one dependent variable, although we can use several independent/predictor variables in the model.

The purpose of this chapter is to discuss the principle conceptual foundations of regression analyses so that readers can have a better understanding of what these analyses can and cannot do and earn a greater appreciation for the types of research questions that such models are suited for. I will provide a few examples with selected (and fabricated) data to help make things more concrete.

Multiple Regression

As noted earlier, independent variables are typically referred to as predictor variables (or covariates, such as in logistic regression), whereas the dependent variable is often referred to as the criterion variable. Multiple regression analysis is much more common and perhaps more appropriate than simple bivariate regression (regression with only one predictor) for one reason: nothing exists in isolation. Many outcomes in life, and in neuropsychology, are multidetermined. We need to account for such interrelatedness and capture which variables, and by how much, are important. This helps to increase the signal to noise ratio in order to discern unique contributions among variables. For example, performance on a test of memory is affected by age, education, sex, fatigue, and attention—to name just a few. Therefore, it would be important and logical to include these multiple predictor variables in a regression analysis. Clearly, sound theoretical reasoning for choosing which predictor variables to include in the analysis is paramount. Including a variable that represents how far a person lives from the testing center solely because such data are accessible is inappropriate.

Methods of Regression Analysis

There are several analytic strategies of regression analysis, each of which is chosen based on the research question. Three of the most common models include: standard regression, hierarchical/sequential regression, and stepwise regression.

Standard Regression

In this mode of analysis, all of the predictor variables are included in one "block." In other words, all predictor variables are entered simultaneously without consideration or concern for their order. (See Fig. 7.1, in which intelligence, executive function, and social support represent predictors in a regression analysis that were entered simultaneously. The dependent variable is coping.)

In the diagram above, intelligence, executive function, and a measure of social support are entered simultaneously to determine which variables are related to coping ability. A theory might be that those who are intelligent and effective problem—solvers and those who perceive strong social and family support cope better with life stressors. The results will not only tell you if the overall regression model is significant, but also which variables predict coping, and which of the three—intelligence, executive function, and social support—are most related to coping.

Hierarchical/Sequential Regression

In this type of regression analysis, the predictors are entered in clusters, or "blocks." The last block contains the variable of chief importance. This method is referred to as a sequential procedure because variables are entered in sequences (e.g., the first block may contain demographic variables such as age and education). This is also referred to as a hierarchical model because the variable under primary consideration is entered last; it is of the utmost importance and placed at the apex of the model. If the last variable remains significant in the final model, then it can be said that it contributes to predicting the criterion variable above and beyond that which is predicted from all other variables that precede it. This is a common method of analysis when examining a test's incremental validity or in covariance analysis in which preceding block are controlled for. Figure 7.2 shows a simplistic model of a hierarchical regression analysis.

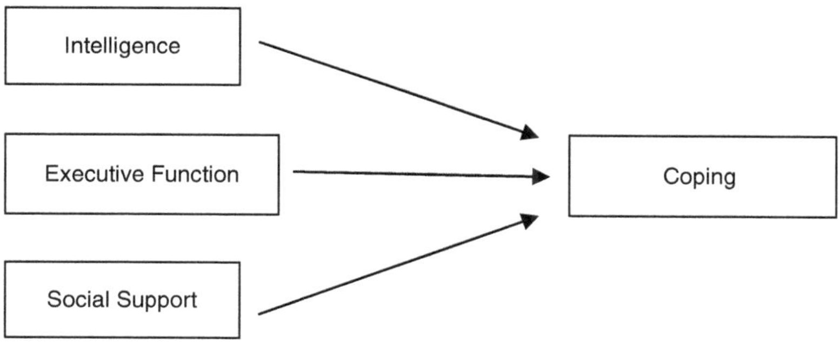

Fig. 7.1 Standard regression analysis. Predictors include: intelligence, executive function, and social support. Coping represents the dependent variable

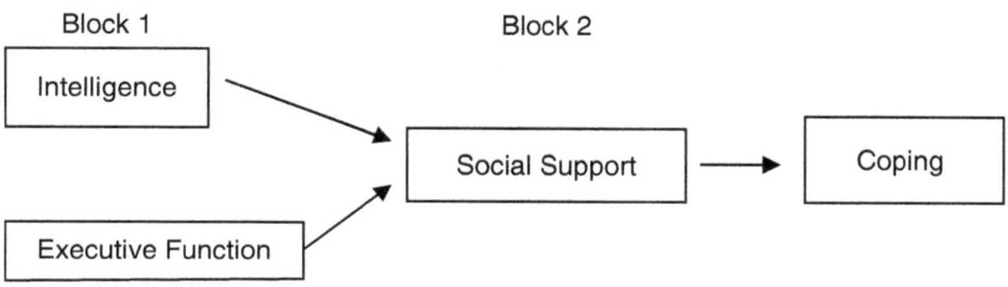

Fig. 7.2 Intelligence and executive function are predictors in block 1. Social support is a predictor and entered into block 2. The criterion variable is coping. Note that the model is attempting to demonstrate that social support explains one's ability to cope above and beyond a person's intellect and executive function

The thrust of the hierarchical model above is that social support is significantly related to coping ability even after controlling for intellectual and cognitive function.

Stepwise Regression

This is also referred to as statistical regression. I like to refer to this as the "click and see" method. All predictors are entered into the analysis. However, the computer determines which variables should remain in the final model. Thus, it is based on statistical criteria rather than theory. Although not considered the true "scientific method," it can help in theory building. This is based on the predictor variable that has the strongest partial correlation [a partial correlation means that the influence of other predictors is partialed out (controlled for) from all other predictors as well as the criterion] *after controlling for all of the variables already in the equation.*

This method has been sharply criticized because it capitalizes on chance. However, it is useful as an exploratory method (e.g., theory building) and in the

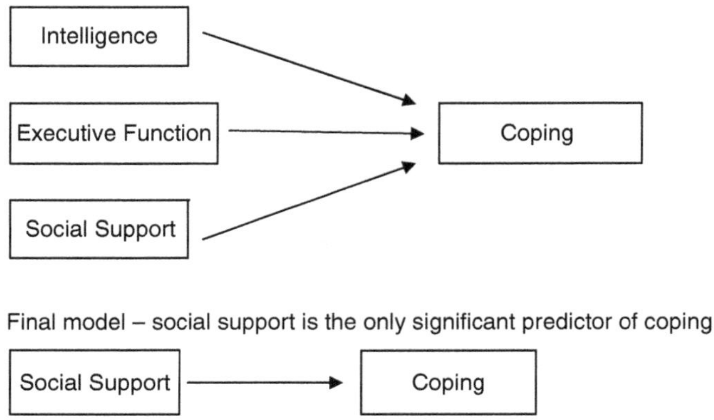

Fig. 7.3 In the first step, all three predictor variables are entered simultaneously

preliminary stages of a nascent and underexplored theory. As Harlow (2005) notes, due to the atheoretical nature of this method, cross-validation and replication are paramount to ensure that the findings are not spurious or sample specific. For example, on a conventional alpha level of 0.05, if 20 variables were examined, it is extremely likely that at least one variable will yield a significant association with the criterion variable merely by chance. In order to ensure the veracity of the preliminary findings, the same regression equation might be used for a separate sample (i.e., cross-validation).

There are a variety of methods within stepwise regression, the most common include forward and backward selection. In backward stepwise regression (see in Fig. 7.3), all variables are entered and only significant variables are retained in the final model. In forward stepwise regression, the model begins without any variables, and each predictor is examined one-by-one. The final model includes only those predictors that are significant.

Before Deciding to Run the Analysis…

Sound theory should always dictate which variables to include in the analysis. Of course, stepwise regression requires that one is more liberal in variable selection as it is atheoretical. In standard and hierarchical analyses, it is not only uncommon to specify which variables to be included, but also to predict which variables will be the most influential, and in which direction the variables are related (i.e., directly or inversely), as in the previous examples.

It is equally important to include covariates in the analysis. Although in methods such as analysis of covariance (ANCOVA) in which the covariate is considered separately, covariates in a regression analysis are included among the predictor variables. Ideally, a covariate is any variable that is related, or varies systematically, with the criterion variable but is not the central focus of the design. For example, age and education are often related to cognitive test performance and are commonly included in analyses. The hope is that the predictor variable is significant in predicting the criterion variable over and above that of the covariates. Or, that even when taking into consideration age and education, particular predictor variables remain significantly related to the criterion.

What Else Can Regression Do?

Another option is to explore interactions among the predictor variables, for example, examining whether age and sex interact to predict performance on a cognitive test. The results might indicate that only older men perform in an unexpected fashion on a test. This would represent an interaction. And, the significance of interactions, just like the main effects of individual variables, can be examined in the analysis.

An interaction term is merely the product of two variables [after each variable has been centered (a deviation score) to avoid collinearity].

Potential Problems for Multiple Regression

A fundamental problem of multiple regression has to do with multicollinearity: when the predictor variables are highly correlated with each other. Generally, a correlation of 0.70 of higher between any pair of predictor variables should raise red flags. Stevens (2002) discussed three drawbacks from multicollinearity:

1. It limits the size of R (the correlation between the predictors and the criterion), because the predictors are empirically and probably conceptually intertwined that they are capturing much of the same variance on the criterion variable. Therefore, it may be counterproductive to include several scores/items that reflect one particular construct—say memory.
2. The importance of a given predictor is muddlers because their individual contributions are difficult to discern because of high correlations.
3. It Increases the variances of the regression coefficients, making the prediction/ regression equation more unstable/precarious.

If there is evidence of multicollinearity, but disposing of one or more variables is implausible, ridge regression (which is beyond the scope of this chapter) may be an appropriate procedure.

Another common pitfall, though not commonly discussed, involves *singularity*. This occurs when one predictor variable in the model is a composite for other variables already included. For example, it would be unwise to include trials one through three of the Hopkins Verbal Learning Test (three variables), in addition to the total recall score, as the total recall score comprises all three learning trials.

Assumptions for Multiple Regression

Several assumptions for regression must be met in order to yield tenable results. These assumptions include normality, linearity, homoscedasticity, and independence of errors. However, other important practical considerations must be taken into consideration, such as the ratio of cases-to-predictor-variables. For example, although too many cases will inevitably result in statistically significant results (but perhaps not clinically significant), too few cases can be equally problematic. If there are too few cases, Tabachnick and Fidell (2001) suggest collapsing a set of predictor variables (into a composite measure) so as not to overload the analysis. For example, instead of including measures of immediate recall, delayed recall, and recognition memory, a general memory composite score might be created that would comprise all three. In addition, outliers, or extreme scores, can be a problem for regression analysis. Scores on neuropsychological measures afford no protection from outliers. Some tests may be more "vulnerable" to outliers, however. For example, reaction time, in which a select few perform uncommonly slow, can skew results. Therefore, examination of outiers (graphically or statistically) can be helpful. Choosing what to do with them if they are present is a different question (e.g., truncating or omitting scores).

If assumptions are not met, transformations are a common techniques to deal with the problem; however, tranformations do not change the relationships among scores but make the data more suitable for analysis. Transformation might include a square root or logarithm of the predictor variables is, and running the analysis with the transformed variables. The difficulty lies in interpreting the results. Normality, linearity, and homoscedasticity can be examined collectively with a residuals analysis (in a scatterplot), which plots the predicted dependent variable scores and the errors of prediction. Measurement reliability is also discussed.

Normality

Residuals should be normally distributed about the predicted dependent variables that is the error between what is observed with the data and which is predictor with the analyses.

Linearity

independent variable, should also have a straignt line relationship with the dependent variables, examining age and memory in a regression, memory should decline. at a constant rate with age.

Homoscedasticity

As described in an earlier Chapter, this dictates that the standard deviations of the errors of the predictors are nearly equal for all predicted dependent variable scores. Thus, the clusters of residuals should have roughly equal widths at each value of the predicted dependent variable. If this assumption is violated (i.e., heteroscedasticity is present), covariates can be included in the analysis.

Residuals about the predicted dependent variable scores should be the same for all the predicted scores. Homoscedasticity means that the variance of errors is the same across all levels of the predictor variable. When the variance of errors differs at different values of the predictor variable, the assumption is violated and the data are considered heteroscedastic. Similar to checking for linearity, examination of the plot of the standardized residuals (errors) by the regression standardized predicted values.

Let's think of performance on any 'fluid' measure over the lifespan. Perhaps if we look at people in their 20s through their 40s, there is perhaps a steady decline in speed of processing. However, as people get older, they encounter more medical problems, etc., and the variability at increasing age is greatest. Some are healthy, some are becoming ill, and some are very ill. Statistically, this would represent a heteroscedastic distribution.

Independence of Errors

This means that the errors of the prediction are independent of one another for example, if an examiner were to learn to score the WAIS-IV, and used each successive participant as a "guinea pig," it might be that due to the larger number of errors earlier on in the learning process, the variability of the test's scores is much greater than toward the latter participants, in which the examiner has become more proficient in scoring the test. This would result in nonindependence of errors.

Likewise, if an examiner were learning to *administer* a test, and made more errors earlier on, performance among participants on this one test is likely to show greater variability initially, only to become more stable and restricted as he/she becomes more skillful.

Measurement Reliability

It is important to ensure that the variables included in the analysis are reliable. A well-established measure (based on previous research) is important. However, it is wise to examine (e.g., via Cronbach's alpha) the reliability of each measure in your analysis. A good rule-of-thumb is that a Cronbach's alpha of 0.7 or greater is acceptable reliability.

Goal and Interpretation of Multiple Regression

The objective of multiple regression is to find a multiple correlation between a newly created linear composite of the predictor variables and the outcome variable. If a test of memory and executive cognition were significantly related to academic achievement, the multiple correlation is a linear composite of the independent variables (memory and executive cognition) and the dependent variable (academic achievement).

Similar to other multivariable and multivariate procedures, the omnibus test statistic in multiple regression does not reveal much information about the individual predictors in the model. If the F-statistic (similar to an ANOVA output; The F-statistic indicates how much of the covariance among the variables is greater than chance relative to the variance within the variables) is significant, then one must look at the signiciance tests (i.e., t-tests) that generally accompany the output and provide for the significance and degree for each predictor (the individual regression weights; B).

Another test statistic to look at is R-squared. This is similar to the r-squared in a bivariate (zero-order) correlation. This tells you both the magnitude of the effect of the relationship between the linear composite of predictor variables and the criterion as well as the shared variance between the linear combinations and the outcome variable. As Cohen (1992) suggested, 0.02, 0.13, and 0.26 represent small, medium, and large effect sizes, respectively.

Researchers often look at the adjusted R-squared value as well. This adjustment takes into consideration possible sample-specific findings, including how many persons and the number of predictors that were in the model. Therefore, the adjusted R is typically a slightly smaller value.

Following Up a Significant Multiple Regression

As I indicated above, once the omnibus test statistic (F-statistic) is significant, individual predictors are examined for significance via t-tests. Because of the family-wise error rate (there are several test statistics within one test), either a Bonferroni correction (dividing an alpha level of 0.05 by the number of statistical tests) or using a more conservative alpha level (e.g., 0.01 or 0.001) is used to guard against a Type I error.

Inspection of the standardized weights will indicate how much a particular predictor variable contributes to the analysis, and how much the predictor variable covaries with the criiterion variable while taking into account the relationships with the other predictor variables.

A standardized regression coefficient is a partial correlation. This represents the effect of a predictor variable after partialing out the effects of all other predictors in the model. The standardized regression weight (Beta weight; B) indicates the relationship between the predictors and the criterion, after recognizing the correlations among the other predictor variables in the equation.

Example of Standard Multiple Regression

We can continue with the above example using intelligence (Full Scale IQ from the WAIS-IV), executive cognition (Towertest; Delis–Kaplan) (Executive Function System) and social support (the Multidimensional Scale of Perceived Social Support; MSPSS) (Zimet, Dahlem, Zimet, & Farley, 1988)) to predict coping (as measured by the Maroof Coping Scale; MCS). The MSPSS has a total of 12 items, with a higher score indicating more perceived social support (a total of 84 points). The MCS is a fictitious scale, but we can assume that it has 15 items and can reach a total of 60 points (i.e., coping extremely well). All predictor variables are entered simultaneously. A selection of the analysis is shown and described below.

From the output seen in Table 7.1, the overall model (ANOVA, $p=0.021$) is significant. Examination of each predictor indicates that FSIQ, DKEFS, and social support are significantly associated with coping. Using the unstandardized coefficients, one can generate a regression (prediction) equation as: $Y=4.605+0.264$ (FSIQ) + 0.546 (DKEFS) + 0.373 (social support), where Y = the value coping. Note that the coefficients in this equation represent the amount of change in coping for each one unit change in the predictor variable. The R-square in the table indicates that about 48% of the variance in coping can be explained by the linear combination of the predictor variables.

Curvilinear Regression

As its name suggests, curvilinear regression is best suited for modeling variables that reflect nonlinear/curvilinear relationships (e.g., a U- or n-shape). Such relationship are not uncommon in neuropsychology. Constant increases or decreases in predictor variables do not necessarily monotonically yield corresponding changes in outcome measures. For example, processing speed generally increases from very early age to the teens and twenties, only to plateau shortly after and then show a decline with advanced age. If one were modeling processing speed as a function of age, a curvilinear regression analysis might be most appropriate.

Table 7.1 Results of omnibus ANOVA and then the significance value of each predictor in a multiple regression analysis

ANOVA					
	Unstand. Coeff.		Stand. Coeff.		
	B	S.E.	beta	t-statistic	p-value
Constant	4.604	2.50	0.588	1.98	0.001
FSIQ	0.264	0.155	0.789	2.4	0.001
DKEFS	0.546	0.254	0.196	1.89	0.017
Social Support	0.373	0.340	0.494	1.94	0.023

$F=3.316, p=0.021$
R-square = 0.475
Note: criterion variable is coping

Take psychopharmacology as another example. A small dosage of an antidepressant may confer little or no benefit (mood improvement). A slightly higher dosage may yield clinically relevant changes in mood. However, an even larger dosage may have either no additional benefit (person's mood may not improve any further), but it might be detrimental. A linear model would not capture this relationship. In fact, a linear model presupposes that the more of the drug the better. This is simply not the case in clinical practice.

Curvilinear regression is a type of polynomial regression. The predictor variables are raised to powers (linear, squared, cubed, quartic, quintic, etc.). To test for nonlinearity (e.g., curvilinear relationships), a hierarchical regression analysis is employed. In the first block, the linear model is tested, and each successive block contains a higher-order polynomial (second block: squared, third block: cubed, etc.). The change in variance with each successive models is examined; the model that best fits the observed data will be the "most" significant.

Summary

The purpose of this chapter was to introduce the reader to regression analysis. Typical research questions that are suitable for linear regression analyses were discussed, as were methods of regression: standard, stepwise, and hierarchical. Several assumptions of regression analysis were considered. Last, brief consideration was provided for nonlinear trends in data, in particular curvilinear regression.

Chapter 8
Binary Logistic Regression

Introduction

Unlike linear regression, which is used to classify or predict values on a continuous variable (e.g., estimated premorbid intelligence), logistic regression attempts to classify or predict a discrete, categorical variable from among continuous and/or discrete predictors, such as whether or not a patient will be successful in cognitive rehabilitation (yes/no; the dichotomous criterion variable) based on premorbid intellectual functioning (the continuous predictor).

Consider a few more examples: Does performance on a test of spatial cognition accurately classify (better than chance) patients with Lewy body dementia and Alzheimer's disease? Do tests of auditory/verbal and spatial/configural learning and memory predict lesions in the right and left hemisphere, respectively? Does performance on a battery of neuropsychological tests predict whether participants are likely to be unemployed, employed, or disabled at a certain time following assessment? Are there particular tests—verbal, visual, etc.—that classify men and women? Do people with a family history of Alzheimer's disease have a greater likelihood of developing the illness than those without a family history?

What all of these examples have in common is that the criterion variable, the dependent or outcome variable, is discrete: Lewy body dementia versus Alzheimer's disease; left versus right hemisphere; unemployed, employed, or disabled; male versus female; disease/no disease.

In binary logistic regression, the outcome variable is dichotomous (hence the term binary, or "involving two"). There is no particular order to the variables, though reference groups are often designated so as to facilitate interpretation of the regression coefficients, and persons functioning as controls often serve this purpose (patients are benchmarked against healthy participants).

There are other forms of logistic regression. Multinomial regression, for example, enables the researcher to classify into more than two groups—normal controls, mild cognitive impairment, and Alzheimer's disease, for example. Other forms of regression are similar, though they have an ordering/ranking to the categories—slow

D.A. Maroof, *Statistical Methods in Neuropsychology: Common Procedures Made Comprehensible*, DOI 10.1007/978-1-4614-3417-7_8,

speed, average speed, fast, for example. In this latter case, ordinal regression would be most appropriate.

For the purpose of this chapter, only binary logistic regression will be discussed. The overarching aim is to provide a concise description of binary logistic regression, to delineate some practical and theoretical issues in its application, and demonstrate how binary logistic regression could be used and interpreted to answer questions in clinical neuropsychological research.

Binary Logistic Regression

Binary logistic regression analysis has become increasingly more common. As mentioned earlier, the dependent (criterion) variable in such an analysis is dichotomous (e.g., male/female, controls/patients, old/young, etc.). Similar to linear regression, the predictors can either be continuous or categorical. However, unlike linear regression whose goal is to predict a score on some outcome measure, the goal of logistic regression is to assess the likelihood of falling into one of the outcome categories based on a set of predictors. For example, logistic regression can be used to assess the odds of a disease given certain characteristics, symptoms, or performances on neuropsychological tests. Are patients who perform poorly when asked to draw a clock face set to a specified time more likely to be "assigned" to patients with Alzheimer's disease or to be placed into the "bin" for "normal" healthy persons? The difference, therefore, between linear and logistic regression, lies in their fundamentally disparate conceptual and practical applications.

Similar to linear regression, the logistic regression model generates an omnibus test statistic that, if significant, examination proceeds to determine which predictors are most strongly related to the outcome.

How Do the Models for Linear and Logistic Regression Differ?

Linear regression attempts to fit a linear (straight line) model to observed data wherein the solution—based on the values of the predictors and the criterion—attempts to minimize the squared distance between the observed values and the predicted values (the residuals); this is how linear regression has gained the sobriquet, "the method of least squares." In plain English, after a number of statistical iterations (attempts at fitting straight lines to the observed data), a straight line that best fits the observed data is selected. This line is such that the distances between the observed values and the straight line (the predicted values) are restrained as best as possible, that is, that it makes the least amount of error (distance) from the observed values. This line, as you may recall, can be expressed as an equation, $y = bx + a$, where y is the outcome variable, b is the slope (the steepness of the line;

how much 'y' will change for every single one point change in x), and 'a' is the constant (how much 'y' would equal should 'x' be zero).

In logistic regression, the intent is not to predict the *value* of the outcome variable (e.g., how someone may score on the Graduate Record Examination), but the prediction is the probability of an event—the outcome—occurring given values on the predictor variables. So, based on an individual's grade point average, one is predicting *not* the GRE score, but perhaps, the likelihood that individual will pass or fail the examination.

Unlike linear regression, logistic regression expresses the regression equation in logarithmic terms to avoid the assumption of linearity. Clearly, the relationship is different and must be modeled accordingly if we are to capture and accurately model nonlinear relationships.

Conceptual Issues in Binary Logistic Regression

Logistic regression attempts to predict the probability that an observation or a score belongs to each of the two groups. The observation is assigned to the group with the higher predicted probability (Wright, 1995). So, if a case were selected at random, and his or her scores were "plugged into" a regression equation, it can tell us to which group or category that person likely belongs. For example, if a patient performed poorly on a recognition memory test, if this score were entered into the regression equation, would the model "predict" that such a score likely comes from patients with Alzheimer's disease rather than healthy persons?

Like any other statistical method, only with serial evaluations and tight methodological control can cause and effect relationships be entertained. Otherwise, the results—significance of correlation coefficients and the odds ratios (both to be discussed shortly)—need to be interpreted cautiously. Try to not forget the deep-rooted apothegm "correlation does not mean causation."

Practical Issues and Assumptions

A major practical issue with logistic regression has to do with the nature of the outcome variables. They must be mutually exclusive and exhaustive, and they cannot be artificially splintered.

As for the first principle, patients either do or do not have a disease. Patients cannot be diagnosed with Alzheimer's disease and at the same time not have Alzheimer's disease. On the other hand, using hypertension and diabetes mellitus as the outcome variables in logistic regression would be inappropriate. These are not mutually exclusive. A patient can both be hypertensive and diabetic.

Unnatural separation of the dependent variable is equally problematic. For example, it would appear ungainly to use a median split on a test of memory, and then classify patients who are impaired and unimpaired. Much more pertinent information would be gleaned by having the memory score remain continuous and then running a linear regression. However, there are times when, due to restricted ranges or markedly skewed distributions collapsing or transforming a variable seems like the most proper solution.

The beauty of a logistic regression is that it does not require typical assumptions of linearity, normality, and/or homoscedasticity. Its counterpart, discriminant function analysis, has many more assumptions than logistic regression.

The most admired and coveted output from logistic regression is the odds ratio. The odds ratio indicates the chance of being in an outcome category given a one-unit change in a predictor variable, after taking into account the other predictor variables in the model. Odds ratios that are greater than one indicate that there is a greater likelihood of falling into the baseline outcome category (e.g., usually normal controls) given an increase of one point in the predictor variable. Odds ratios less than one indicate that there is less likelihood of falling into the reference/outcome category when the value for a predictor is increased by one point.

Interpreting Logistic Regression

Like linear (or curvilinear) regression, there is an omnibus test statistic to determine whether the overall model is significant. In linear regression, examination of the F-statistic from an ANOVA is examined, whereas in logistic regression, a chi square statistic tells you whether the model and its predictors are significantly greater than the constant alone.

In addition to the constant, a regression coefficient for each predictor variable is generated. You can then use individual values (e.g., scores on the predictor variables) to compute on an individual basis the predicted probability of being assigned into a specific group.

Interpreting logistic regression can involve either examination of the odds ratios, which is the chance of being in the outcome category given one unit change in the predictor variable after taking into account all other predictors in the model, or with individual coefficients. However, odds ratios generally provide the most interesting information with regard to relationships among variables. A brief description of odds ratios is in order.

Odds Ratios

There are a number of concepts in the medical and social sciences that leave us feeling bewildered. This is because the nuanced language and subtle gradations in meaning (as well as the convoluted mathematical formulae) make such efforts quite challenging. However, differentiating between two commonly mistaken statistics—relative risk and odds ratios—is in order. These values are calculated differently, their meanings are not equivalent, and they require different interpretations.

Relative risk is a ratio of probabilities of two events. For example, women's risk of developing multiple sclerosis is two times that of men. So the risk of developing multiple sclerosis for women is relative to the same risk for men. For example, if the probability of developing multiple sclerosis in women is 2%, and for men it is 1%, then using the simple ratio of the probability of two events (2% for women/1% for men=2). This is because the probability of the first event (women developing multiple sclerosis) is divided by the probability of the second event (men developing multiple sclerosis).

The term "odds" is both conceptually and mathematically distinct from relative risk. Odds is a ratio of the probability that an event will happen divided by the probability of the event not occurring. So we are asking, how likely will an event occur (e.g., that someone will develop multiple sclerosis) in comparison to the likelihood that the event will not occur? This is *not* the same as an odds ratio, which goes a little bit farther.

An odds ratio is a comparison of an event (e.g., diagnosis) occurring in two different groups. The ratio (in odds ratio) is simply the odds for the first group and the odds for the second group. As Wright says, an odds tells you how much more likely it is that an observation is a member of the target group rather than a member of the other group.

For example, let's say that the likelihood of being cognitively normal (whatever that means) for persons under 40 years of age is about 50%. Therefore, the odds for this group are 1 (50% of getting an illness/50% of not getting an illness). Therefore, the persons in this group are equally likely to be diagnosed with a given illness (or not). However, for persons over 40 years of age, the chance of remaining healthy is about 20%. The odds for a person over 40 is thus 20%/80% (80% chance of not getting an illness), or 0.25. This means that for every one person who remains healthy, there are four people who develop an illness (1/0.25=4).

This does not mean that people under 40 are four times more likely to remain healthy. However, based on relative risk (a ratio of probabilities), a person under 40 years of age is 2.5 times more likely to remain healthy (50%/20%). On the other hand, we can say the persons under 40 have four times the odds as those over 40 of remaining healthy.

For logistic regression, the odds remains the same for all levels of the groups with one unit change in predictor variable.

As noted earlier, examination of individual predictors indicates which variables are significantly related to the outcome. Positive values mean the odds increases as the value of the predictor increases, whereas negative values signify the predicted odds descreases as the predictor value increases.

Examples of Logistic Regression in Neuropsychological Research

Example 1: Errors in Scoring Neuropsychological Batteries

In this example research question, we would like to determine whether scoring errors from neuropsychological tests can predict whether someone who score the battery is either a graduate student (intern or fellow) or a neuropsychologist.

Errors are an inevitable part of research, clinical practice, and life. Neuropsychological testing—in particular, scoring—is not invulnerable to errors. For one, we are human. However, the process involved in scoring neuropsychological measures involves maneuvering a plethora of tests, rifling through a host of test manuals, calculating standard scores [some of which need to be reversed in value because they are timed measures or they are errors, therefore, larger raw scores (slower time and more mistakes, respectively) indicate poorer performance] and percentiles from disparate normative samples, and imputing the information into a data table. If anyone can navigate all these steps without believing they have made a single error, then, they just made another error!

For the sake of this example, suppose we used archival data to comb through a select group of patients who underwent neuropsychological testing (at any given clinic, and perhaps, with the same battery of tests). The researchers select a number of charts comprising a battery of neuropsychological tests. They tally each error that they find, as well as whether the scoring involved either a student or a faculty member. For purposes of this example, errors are collapsed into one category, and involve a variety of clerical errors (e.g., tallying the number or items incorrectly on a test, or miscalculating a standard score). In the database, each participant (either student of faculty member) represents a case, and, the number of errors represents the dependent variable. Thus, so far we have two columns: one for group (student/faculty), and the other for errors (a quantitative value that ranges anywhere from zero errors and beyond). The ratio of the number of errors per group member based on the number of indices he or she scored should be considered (to keep everything on an even playing field). However, we can assume that each case in this study scored the same number of tests. Therefore, we can use the raw scores.

First, let's examine why this question would fit into a binary logistic regression model. The predictor (independent variable) is continuous: the number of errors. And, the outcome measure is dichotomous (and mutually exclusive: one cannot be a student and a neuropsychologist concurrently). Our goal is to see, given the number of errors, whether a particular group is more likely to make errors. And, given the number of errors on any given battery, can we predict whether the battery was more likely scored by either a student or a faculty member? The model will also tell us the overall accuracy of classification.

Other than the number of errors, there are a host of factors that can explain or contribute to classifying group membership. Therefore, we might want to include one or more covariates into the analysis. The goal of doing so is to ensure that, most things being roughly equal, can we attribute any differences to the training status of the participants, rather than to other possible factors. We could include age and education. But let's stop and think for one second. Both age and education are likely to be intertwined with training status. That is, faculty members are likely older, and because they *are* faculty members, their education levels are higher. Therefore, it would be inappropriate to include any one of these variables as a covariate.

There are other possible confounding variables. We might want to include sex as a covariate (if we were to have a sufficient number of participants). We can use a standard (enter method) binary logistic regression in which both sex (a dichotomous

Table 8.1 Results of binary logistic regression analysis

Variable	b	SE	P	Odds ratio	CI for odds ratio
Sex	0.87	0.75	0.09	1.34	0.74–1.44
Errors	0.97	0.82	0.03	3.21	2.45–3.89

Note: outcome variable = student/faculty. CI = confidence interval

predictor) and errors are entered as predictors (covariates) into one block and have training status represent the dichotomous outcome variable.

For interpretive purposes, let us say that we have dummy coded students 0 and faculty members 1. As for sex, we can dummy code males 0, and females 1. Dummy coding does not convey any quantitative information about the variables themselves. In other words, males being coded as 0 does not mean that they matter less than females who are coded 1. The purpose of knowing how the dichotomous variables are coded is to aid in interpretation of the coefficients. Also, although it does not make intuitive sense to predict whether someone is a student or faculty member based on their sex. Including sex in the model will help us answer the question, irrespective of sex of the individual who scored the testing, can we still determine whether either group is more likely to have made errors?

The sign (positive or negative) of the regression coefficients indicates in what way a predictor variable is related to the outcome variable. The results of this experiment are provided below.

Let us first assume that the omnibus test statistic is significant. We can therefore proceed to examine the individual predictors in the model (as seen in Table 8.1.). From the selected output above, it is apparent that sex is not significantly associated with predicting training status. However, this variable is essentially serving as a covariate, and is not the primary focus of this study.

The results in the last row (errors) tell us this variable is a significant predictor of training status ($p = 0.03$). Interpreting the odds ratio, then, informs us that for every additional error (for every one unit increase in the predictor variable), the odds of being classified as a student (the reference category) is more than three times as likely (odds ratio = 3.21). As the confidence interval for this odds ratio does not encompass 1 (one means that there is no relation between errors and training status). Keep in mind that I have not included the omnibus test statistic (chi square statistic) to determine whether the model is significant and in fact better at predicting group membership than the constant in the equation.

Example 2: Do Case Conferences Increase the Accuracy of a Diagnosis Above Individually Independent Diagnosis?

Clinical case conferences are a wonderful avenue for eliciting feedback from others on a particular case. It helps gain perspective about a case, and is especially useful in ambiguous or rare presentations. One can argue that the use of clinical case

Table 8.2 Results of binary logistic regression analysis

Variable	b	SE	P	Odds ratio	CI for odds ratio
Age	0.67	0.65	0.21	1.14	0.78–1.41
Experience	0.77	0.72	0.10	1.21	0.45–1.05
Group	0.90	0.75	0.02	1.34	1.09–1.44
Group x Experience	0.87	0.85	0.11	1.24	0.74–1.44

Note: outcome variable = accuracy of diagnosis (accurate or inaccurate). Group = individual or clinical case conference. Group x experience = interaction

conferences improves the accuracy of diagnosing because, well, two (or more) heads are greater than one. That being said, we might argue that diagnosing independently (without others' feedback) is more prone to inaccuracy.

The purpose of this experiment is to determine whether diagnoses made at an individual level are any different, or accurate, than diagnoses made with the help of a clinical case conference.

One hundred clinical neuropsychologists are selected for this study. Fifty neuropsychologists are provided with 75 cases and are asked to render a diagnosis. The other fifty neuropsychologists are provided with the same 75 clinical cases. However, in the latter group, after they make a diagnosis, they attend a clinical case conference. After presenting the case, they are offered feedback from among a larger group of neuropsychologists. They may choose to relinquish, refine, or redefine the diagnosis based on the information provided from others.

Of note, all 75 cases were independently diagnosed (independent from any of the neuropsychologists, including those in the clinical case conference).

Again, let's examine why this research question is appropriate for analysis with binary logistic regression. First, our predictor variable, individual versus clinical case conference (a dichotomous predictor variable), is appropriate in a regression analysis. Second, the outcome variable, whether or not the diagnosis is correct, is dichotomous. So far, so good? This is entirely suitable for a binary logistic regression analysis.

The goal of this study is to determine whether clinicians who diagnose independently are equally accurate in diagnosing. We have to dummy code both the predictor and the outcome variable. As for the predictor variable, the individual diagnosis = 0. For the outcome variable, the incorrect diagnosis = 0.

Before we decide to run the analysis. It might be interesting to look at additional predictors. Age and years of experience of the clinicians' (those making the final diagnosis, not necessarily the clinicians in the case conference, although that may also be considered). We might also be interested as to whether years of experience and the primary predictor variable (individual versus case conference diagnosis) interact. Our a priori hypothesis might be that those with the most experience who are receiving feedback from others will be the most accurate in diagnosing the patients. The results from the analysis are provided down below.

There are a number of things to examine in Table 8.2. Keep in mind, we can assume that the overall omnibus test statistic was significant. Inspection of the p-values tells us that age, experience (or the interaction between the two) are significant. However, holding all of those variables equivalent, we see that group (whether the diagnosis was rendered on an individual or group (case conference)) basis was significantly related to the accuracy of the diagnosis.

The difference between this example and the prior example is that this time we have a categorical/dichotomous predictor as opposed to a continuous predictor (and we have an interaction term, but this is insignificant).

The take home message is that irrespective of age or years of experience, clinicians who are involved in a case conference are more likely to render an accurate diagnosis than are individuals who diagnose independently. The odds ratio for clinical case conference when age and years of experience are adjusted for, the odds of accurate diagnosis are 1.34 times greater for those with clinical case than for individuals.

Summary

The purpose of this chapter was to describe binary logistic regression. This model allows for examining the association of continuous or categorical predictor variables and a dichotomous outcome variable. Similarities and differences between linear and logistic regression were discussed, as well as some of the practical and conceptual principles of logistic regression. Understanding the output of logistic regression, including the significance of individual predictors as well as the odds ratio was discussed. Two simple examples using binary logistic regression were provided.

Chapter 9
Multivariate Analysis of Variance

Introduction

Multivariate analysis of variance (MANOVA) is an omnibus procedure that allows for the contemporaneous analysis of more than one dependent variable. Dependent variables are the outcome variables, or criteria, of a research design. Performance on neuropsychological tests—memory scores, reaction time, processing speed, the number of words generated on tests of word fluency—can all serve as dependent variables. Interestingly, these dependent variables are often reversed and used as independent variables, or predictors, when interpreting the results of a significant MANOVA. And, scores on neuropsychological tests occasionally serve as independent variables in their own right. For example, one can empirically (e.g., median split) dichotomize performance on any one measure, say processing speed, and then compare persons who are "slow" and "fast" (the independent, or grouping variable) on a number of other dependent variables.

Within any statistical design, it is the experimenter's hypotheses that guide what side of the equation the variables lay. The variables themselves have no bearing on whether they are the predictors or the predicted. Similarly, the scale of measurement (i.e., nominal, ordinal, interval, or ratio) does not necessarily equate with the nature of the variable (see Table 9.1). For example, one can use memory scores as continuous variables (which would qualify as an interval or ratio level of measurement), or define a cut-off (e.g., 1.5 standard deviations below the mean) to define those with impaired and intact memory, and then separate groups based on this created (nominal/categorical) variable. It is the intent (and ingenuity) of the researcher that guides the statistical model, which is "custom made" for a particular study and hypothesis.

The dependent variables used in MANOVA must be continuous variables. That is, they must reflect gradations in test performance—and hence, the inherent ability that they reflect—rather than discrete variables, such as sex or whether someone is a democrat or republican. As I mentioned above, the ability to interpret the results of a significant MANOVA often involves reversing the independent and

D.A. Maroof, *Statistical Methods in Neuropsychology: Common Procedures Made Comprehensible*, DOI 10.1007/978-1-4614-3417-7_9,

Table 9.1 Examples of commonly examined variables used on different scales of measurement

Nominal/Categorical	Interval/Ratio
1. Left/right handed	Edinburgh handedness inventory
2. Depressed/not depressed	Beck depression inventory
3. High/low blood pressure	Systolic/diastolic values
4. Good memory/bad memory	Raw scores on test
5. Positive/negative symptoms	SAPS and SANS*

Note: SAPS Scale for the assessment of positive symptoms (Andreasen, 1984), *SANS* Scale for the assessment of negative symptoms (Andreasen, 1983)

dependent variables and re-running a mathematically homogeneous, albeit, seemingly disparate, analysis. Specifically, after a significant MANOVA, the test scores are used to classify (or predict) the grouping variable. For example, if one establishes that mean differences exist on memory scores between patients and healthy persons, the next step would involve examining not only which of the memory scores e.g., recall or recognition are significant and contribute to classifying the two groups, but also, which scores are most influential. This is achieved with common statistical tests such as logistic regression or discriminant function analysis, the latter of which is mathematically identical to MANOVA. However, there are other procedures for examining a significant MANOVA, including running separate univariate analyses of variance (ANOVAs) on each dependent variable, but this, as well as some variations of the ANOVA procedure, is theoretically unsatisfying for reasons that will soon be discussed. Using logistic regression or discriminant function analysis allows for the simultaneous inclusion of test scores, similar to the MANOVA, and establishes which of the dependent variables, and in what particular weighted combination, best classify and separate group membership.

The purpose of this chapter is to discuss the advantages and disadvantages of MANOVA as well as the assumptions of using this procedure. An example of using and interpreting a MANOVA in neuropsychological research is also provided. I am hopeful that after reading this chapter you will be able to read relevant journal articles with a greater appreciation and understanding of MANOVAs. You should be able to understand why researchers chose to run a MANOVA among their analyses and the purposes and limitations of their follow-up procedures and interpretations. In addition, you will no longer be ill-equipped to render opinions on the appropriateness, or lack thereof, of other researchers' use of such procedures.

As in all other chapters of this book, the emphasis rests on the *concrete* use and interpretation of MANOVAs, rather than on the mathematics behind this procedure. Providing such wiredrawn information is neither the purpose of this chapter nor of this book. My giving short shrift to the math behind statistical techniques is not intended to convey its insignificance.

There is also no emphasis or even discussion on how the MANOVA, or any other statistical procedure, is run in statistical software packages. Such "point and click" methods can be figured out rather easily. There certainly is no shortage of books on the matter.

MANOVA Basics

MANOVA helps us examine statistically what we typically observe in the real world: the effects of one or more variables on a number of outcomes. For example, if you were to examine the effect of exercise on only one variable, say, weight, you would be neglecting several other very important aspects of health. Physical variables such as heart rate, blood pressure, and body mass index, as well as psychological variables, such as self-confidence, depression, motivation, are all likely affected, or perhaps, mediate or moderate, healthy behaviors. A MANOVA would take into consideration several conceptually or empirically related variables and thus provide for a more comprehensive, and generally more accurate, depiction of reality. While several ANOVAs—examining each physical or psychological variable in isolation—would be feasible, they would not capture the interrelationships among the variables. However, one would not be advised to include both physical and psychological variables in one analysis. Since psychological and physical variables are fundamentally disparate provinces of human experience—physical versus the social sciences—they might best be examined with two separate MANOVAs.

In neuropsychological studies, related variables can be "plugged" into a MANOVA. As mentioned, it is often best to choose variables that are similar either conceptuality or entirically. For example, from a large battery of neuropsychological tests, one might include scores from the Hopkins Verbal Learning Test and the Brief Visuospatial Memory Test, immediate, delayed recall, and recognition scores (which is a total of six dependent variables) to one MANOVA. They share one overarching conceptual framework: memory.

It is not uncommon for researchers to unload all available test scores into one omnibus analysis. The problem with this poses both theoretical and empirical pitfalls. It betrays a fundamental misunderstanding of the purposes of statistical analyses, which are to be used as tools for examining hypotheses. At times, such methods are sought to explore clinical hunches, amorphous visions, and/or inchoate ideas. These methods should not serve as a catchall for all available variables. The problem often becomes most conspicuous, and cumbersome, when one is left in the unwieldy position of "retrofitting" the results to fit a newly minted, and often tenuous, theory. This adds nothing to the field of neuropsychology other than fodder for journal groups!

Experimental Versus NonExperimental Designs

In experimental paradigms, the effects of manipulation of the independent variables on the dependent variables are examined. The dependent variables therefore *depend* on the level of the independent variable. That is, if there is an effect on the dependent variables after manipulating the independent variables, the outcome variables should be systematically altered with those manipulations.

It is more common to have nonexperimental, non-manipulated, groups. In this case, one simply examines the mean differences of test scores between groups. Generally, whether or not the analysis is based on experimental or nonexperimental designs, one can still describe, interpret, or explain based on the results. The ability to infer cause and effect, however, is stymied when using non-experimental designs, as one has not established sufficient control and manipulation of the variables to proffer such bold and decisive conclusions. So, without manipulation of the independent variable (s), researchers must rely on descriptive rather than inferential conclusions.

Reasons for MANOVA

While several ANOVAs can be used to examine multiple dependent variables, they are often incapable at handling the interrelationships among the dependent variables. In fact, the dependent variables should be correlated and share a common conceptual meaning. MANOVAS have an advantage over univariate tests. Differences between groups are generally not isolated to a single test score, or a circumscribed neuropsychological function. Therefore, one can yield a more exhaustive and detailed description of the phenomena under interest when multiple outcome variables are included in the analysis.

Give Me a Good Reason!

Stevens (2002) delineated four *statistical* reasons for choosing a MANOVA over the use of multiple univariate analyses:

1- To constrain Type I error
2- So as not to neglect the interrelationships among the dependent variables/avoiding conceptual overlap
3- To capture the best set of variables that best differentiate the groups; any variable in isolation may not be "detected"
4- To avoid a "canceling out effect"

Type I Error

Type I error is the probability of finding a statistical significance in your analyses, when in fact, there is no such difference in reality. This can have very important clinical implications. In fact, several diagnostic screening tests in medicine prefer to misdiagnose (false positive) than to miss a diagnosis.

If you were to use multiple ANOVAs, there is an approximately 5% chance for 40 each analysis that you will generate a false positive, or type I error. If you were to run a series of ANOVAs, clearly, the likelihood that one of the significant findings in your study is a byproduct of chance, rather than a veritable significance, is quite high. A MANOVA uses an overall alpha level in its main analysis. This way, no matter how many dependent variables are included in the analysis, the probability of a Type I error remains at 5% (the alpha level).

Corrections can be applied to the alpha level should one choose to run several ANOVAs. The most commonly used approach is the Bonferroni correction. Simply put, one divides the number of tests by the alpha level. So for example, if you were to run four ANOVAs, you would set the critical level for significance at 0.0125 (0.05/4). The problem with this method is that it is perhaps overly conservative and greatly reduces power. In fact, the Holms-Sequential Bonferroni procedure (Holm, 1979), which is not very common, uses a sequential method of reducing the alpha level so as to protect against a Type I error. Specifically, following a series of univariate tests, the tests are ordered from the smallest to the largest p-value. The test with the lowest probability value is examined with the Bonferroni correction involving all tests. The second lowest p-value is test with a Bonferroni correction after removing one test (and hence, a smaller denominator). This process continues (removing two tests, etc.). This approach overcomes the drawbacks of the conventional Bonferroni approach and uses a less conservative approach, thereby minimizing the risk of Type I error.

Avoiding Conceptual Overlap

Using a linear combination of dependent variables to compare groups is often more sensitive, and more appropriate, particularly in neuropsychology. Using a clinical example, suppose you were referred a patient: a 74-year-old gentleman who reports recent word-finding difficulties, memory problems, and episodes of topographical disorientation. His medical history is relatively unremarkable, and he has a very strong family history of Alzheimer's disease. On neuropsychological testing, he is not oriented to time (misstates the year), shows poor acquisition and retention on memory tests, his semantic fluency is much poorer than his phonemic fluency, and his rendering of a clock face with the hands set at a specified time is deficient. Collectively, most neuropsychologists would agree that this represents a prototypical case of Alzheimer's disease. We base this not only on the context of this man's history—both personal and familial—but also on the pattern of test scores.

Think of this same concept, but in research. If you were to compare persons with Alzheimer's disease (perhaps diagnosed through another method so as to avoid circularity) to healthy elderly persons, a MANOVA would be best able to capture the linear composites of test scores—a better reflection of some underlying construct, the linchpin that links these variables, is clinically meaningful.

For example, we often think of persons with Alzheimer's disease as showing a breakdown in semantic knowledge, which is why we often see profiles as I have just mentioned, in particular poor clock drawing, and semantic fluency, and memory.

Avoid Misidentifying Differences and Conceptual Overlap

The problems inherent in running a number of univariate analyses include using outcome measures that share some level of conceptual overlap. Examining test scores in isolation may fail to identify genuine differences between groups. However, a MANOVA compares vectors of means, and captures the conceptual similarities among test scores. It therefore may be more likely (sensitive) to detect differences between groups. In other words, this may reduce the risk of Type II errors (saying differences are not significant when in actuality they are).

Cancelling Out Effect

A MANOVA may be able to detect differences that a univariate ANOVA may fail to discern. Therefore, choosing a MANOVA over an ANOVA may minimize the risk of a type II error.

Using composite scores in analyses may dissemble veritable differences between groups, so analyzing individual scores from tests (subtests) may yield more profitable results. For example, the Repeatable Battery for the Assessment of Neuropsychological Status (Randolph, 1998) consists of 12 subtests, which yields five indices (and a total "global impairment index"). Of the five indices, the Language Index comprises Picture Naming and Semantic Fluency. If a total composite score were used to compare groups, it may not detect differences between these distinct domains of cognitive function (fluency and naming). Perhaps one group will have performed poorly on naming, the other group on semantic fluency. However, each group's low scores are offset by high scores on the other test, rendering the composite scores roughly equivalent. Separating these performances—examining the performance on both Picture Naming and Semantic Fluency representing two dependent variables—a MANOVA would discern such differences.

Similarly, Delayed Memory on the RBANS comprises verbal (list recall and recognition, and story recall) and visual (figure recall) memory—generating a composite delayed recall score. If these composite scores were used in analyses, rather than examining each as a variable in their own right, then subtle, perhaps lateralizing (right versus left hemisphere involvement) information would not be apparent.

Assumptions of MANOVA

Like all statistical tests, there are assumptions, both statistical and methodological, which can affect the results and ultimately the inferences of the analysis. There are three principle assumptions of MANOVA: multivariate normality, homogeneity of covariance matrices, and independence of observations.

Multivariate Normality

By now, you are familiar with univariate normality. When running univariate tests, such as t-tests or ANOVAs, examining the distribution of each independent variable (and within each group) is second-nature. So, if you were comparing men and women on a memory test, you would examine the distribution of memory scores for men and women separately. Univariate normality requires that the dependent variables are normally distributed. There are statistical and graphical methods for examining univariate normality. For example, in an independent measures t-test, by default, programs such as SPSS will often generate the test statistic, and its probability value, for Levene's test. There are also Probability Plots. In these plots, data are benchmarked against a theoretical normal distribution in such a way that the points should form an approximate the shape of this line of a predicted normal distribution. Thus, departures from this straight line indicate departures from normality. Univariate normality is often a prerequisite, and sometimes considered a substitute, for multivariate normality. However, such procedures fail to detect violations of the assumption of multivariate normality. For example, if you were to examine a large database, a 22-year-old in the sample would not raise any red flags. Likewise, a person who has a very low score on a memory test would go unnoticed. However, a 22-year-old who performs poorly on a memory test is unusual. Testing for univariate normality would fail to identify such violations.

Multivariate normality is more complex because it involves examining all dependent variables simultaneously. Not only must you meet the assumptions of univariate normality, but any linear composite of the dependent variables must be normally distributed as well. Also, as Stevens (2002) indicates, all subets of the set of variables must have multivariate normal distributions: all pairs of variables must be bivariate normal so that for correlated variables, the scatterplots for each pair will be elliptical.

Homogeneity of Covariance Matrices

Homogeneity essentially means similar in kind, or of uniform nature. Covariance matrices refer to whether items cluster together. Therefore, this assumption requires that the variances—or the variability among test scores—are the same across all levels of the dependent variable. It also requires that the correlations between any two dependent variables are the same in all groups. This is particularly concerning if the sample sizes differ across groups.

Box's M Test (Box, 1949) is a statistical means for determining whether this assumption is met. A non-significant Box's M Test indicates the variance-covariance matrices are the same.

Follow-Up Analyses

After running a MANOVA, and examining the significance value of whichever test statistic you so choose, a significant value indicates that the linear combination of means (the vector of means) between the groups differs. However, it does not tell you where and in what combination. There are many procedures for detecting which dependent variables are significant. I will discuss a few here: multiple univariate tests and logistic regression (Huberty & Morris 1989).

Multiple Univariate Analyses

A common, albeit an often problematic, approach to follow up a significant MANOVA is use of univariate tests—t-tests or ANOVAs, for example—for each dependent variable to determine which variable, or variables, is significant between the groups. The rationale for such an approach hinges on the staunch, yet erroneous conviction that using a MANOVA procedure is only used to reduce the risk of Type I error. Therefore, if the MANOVA is significant, running separate univariate analyses would not undermine the utility of subsequent analyses, offering more solace in the possibility that significant findings are not necessarily spurious.

The problem, though, in using several univariate analyses is that it neglects to capture the interrelationships among the dependent variables. Similar to a factorial analysis of variance, where examination of effect of each independent variable on the dependent variable, you can also examine the interaction between two or more independent variables on the dependent variable. Running univariate analysis separately for each independent variable would fail to capture the synergistic effect of the independent variables.

Binary Logistic Regression (or Discriminant Function Analysis)

These procedures are very similar. Discriminant function analysis is mathematically identical to MANOVA and requires several assumptions. Logistic regression on the other hand, requires far fewer assumptions. Both procedures attempt to classify/predict a dichotomous variable (e.g., male/female, controls/Alzheimer's disease) from either continuous or categorical independent variables. This is the exact reverse of a MANOVA in which you are looking at mean differences on test scores between groups. In logistic regression, we are seeing if the test scores can classify group membership; the test scores from the MANOVA, once the dependent variables, are now the independent (covariates) variables.

The advantages of using this procedure is that one can simultaneously examine the weight of each variable on maximizing group classification. This is done simply by looking at which variables remain significant in the analysis, and then, examining which of the standardized weights (among the predictors) is largest. This indicates which of the variables best maximizes group classification while controlling for all other variables in the model.

A General Example Using MANOVA in Neuropsychology

Let's suppose you were interested in studying cognitive performance among coffee drinkers. You randomly assign two groups: one group is assigned to drink no coffee, another group one cup of coffee, and a third, two cups of coffee. A neuropsychological battery is administered that includes: verbal and visual learning and memory, executive function, spatial cognition, and motor and processing speed. Typically, neuropsychological batteries yield numerous scores. Running several analyses of variance (ANOVAs) would be possible, but not ideal. In fact, as many neuropsychological tests are generally correlated, but do not necessarily assess the same cognitive domain, a MANOVA would be used where the dependent variables—the raw scores from the neuropsychological tests—were entered into one comprehensive analysis. This way, we can determine whether there are mean differences among the groups of coffee drinkers on any one dependent variable, such as processing speed, or on some combination of dependent variables. Our overall test statistic, of which there are many which will be discussed shortly, yielded by a MANOVA will simply tell us whether or not there is significance among the groups. If there is no significance, there is nothing more to do. However, if an omnibus test statistic is significant, we must determine where and what differentiates the groups (Table 9.2).

Examination of Table 9.3—with selected output from one of four test statistics—indicates a significant omnibus MANOVA. Follow-up analysis with logistic regression, as seen in Table 9.4, indicates that the Grooved Pegboard Test and the Symbol Digit Modalities Test are significant predictors of whether someone is a coffee drinker. The positive values for the coefficients (i.e, B-column) indicate that as one proceeds from the reference group (non-coffee drinkers) to the reference group (coffee drinkers), scores become higher (i.e., worse performance).

The next step would clearly involve interpretation. Based on this simplistic example, the common denominator for the Grooved Pegboard Test and Symbol Digit Modalities Test seems to be motor speed. The results, therefore, suggest that coffee drinkers perform more slowly on tests that require rapid motor speed.

Table 9.2 Descriptive statistics for tests

	Coffee drinkers	Non-coffee drinkers
Grooved pegboard test	65 s	54 s
Grooved pegboard test	56	47
PASAT	43	43

Note: PASAT = Paced auditory serial addition test: For the PASAT, values represent the mean number correct. For the Symbol Digit Modalities Test, values represent mean number completed in 90 s

Table 9.3 Selected output of MANOVA

	Value	F	Significance
Wilks' Lambda	0.34	623.4	0.000

Note: Independent variable = coffee/no coffee. Dependent variables = Grooved Pegboard Test, Symbol Digit Modalities Test, Paced Auditory Serial Addition Test

Table 9.4 Logistic regression: Follow-up analysis

	B	Sig.	Odds ratio
Constant			
GPT	2.3	0.001	1.44
SDMT	3.1	0.001	1.40
PASAT	0.7	0.280	1.01

Summary

This chapter described MANOVA at conceptual and practical levels. First, the purposes of using MANOVAs were reviewed, which included the simultaneous analysis of two or more conceptually related dependent variables. Next, important reasons for choosing to run a MANOVA were examined, including dealing with Type I error, so as not to neglect the interrelatedness among variables, and avoiding 'canceling out' effects. Assumptions of using a MANOVA were considered: multivariate normality and homogeneity of covariance matrices. Follow-up analyses for determining which variables best distinguish between groups was assessed, including ANOVAs, and binary logistic regression, as well as the limitations and illusions of using certain follow-up paradigms. Finally, a brief case description of MANOVA used in neuropsychology was outlined.

Chapter 10
Reading Critically the Research Literature

Introduction

Everyone is a critic! But, that's just fine. It is in our nature to evaluate and pass judgment. Without this inherent ability, we would live mundane lives, we would never improve as people or as societies, and we would never argue with our significant others about whether wearing black shoes with brown pants is a mortal sin.

The ability to critique research articles affords similar privileges, although, it might be difficult to empirically differentiate good from bad fashion sense, but not impossible! We have by now grown accustomed to reading books, articles, research papers, and the like. However, we generally do not question the veracity of what we read. And, reading and understanding are not interdependent entities.

There can also exist quite a large discrepancy between experience (exposure, perhaps) and skill. This holds very true for reading the neuropsychology literature. You have likely read a number of articles by now, but there is a difference between quantity and quality. The quality I am referring to entails how much one is able to extrapolate from an article, and being able to discriminate between good and bad work. It is important to develop the skills to be able to discern valued research for two main reasons: We base many of our clinical decisions from research; and, it teaches us more about the instruments clinicians use and the limitations of clinical practice.

This Is Nothing New!

You are already well versed in critiquing pretty much everything you encounter in life on a daily basis. The coffee you had this morning might not have tasted right, so you asked our favorite barista for a new cup of hot coffee. You make adjustments to your pants when they seem not to be fitting right, and you incessantly vet presidential candidates. The point is that we base the majority of our decisions, be they personal, professional, or political, from constant vigilance and judgment.

D.A. Maroof, *Statistical Methods in Neuropsychology: Common Procedures Made Comprehensible*, DOI 10.1007/978-1-4614-3417-7_10,

Our decisions and appraisals are arrived at following a period after which we have weighed the available evidence and determined what we think is the most reasonable conclusion.

By now, you should have an idea of what I am getting at. The ability and tendency for us to discern imprecisions and inaccuracies helps us avoid adversity. These adversities can range from subtle embarrassments to tremendous professional blunders.

Detecting and correcting imperfections does not make us obstinate, fastidious, or arrogant. Rather, it makes us skillful and astute; attributes that are often rewarded in science. If anything, this skill offers us greater awareness of what we read, write, and say.

Anyone can read through an article, but not everyone has the scientific acumen to spot errors. Not everyone can discern nuanced language chosen by the authors that transforms an edible dessert into an inedible desert. It takes skill to distinguish incongruencies between study hypotheses and study design, between study results and study inferences, and between a study's emphasis and its often tenuous and ill-conceived title. Accuracy, precision, and concision on paper reflect the clarity of one's thinking, the strength of one's ideas, and the conviction of one's principles.

But It's Published Work

It is all too easy to be allured by the authoritative appeal of published work (after all, you are reading this book, aren't you?). However, not all research should be treated the same. It is your responsibility to determine whether the information you read is something you do or do not agree with. And, whichever of two positions you have co-opted, you should be able to state with steadfast conviction why you have done so. If you are asked why you believe using reliable change indices in clinical practice is a suspect you should be able to offer a cogent rationale of why you hold credence in such views.

In reading research articles, it is also for you to determine whether the hypotheses generated make sense, whether the methods and procedures for testing those hypotheses are sound, and whether the discussion section is accurate and reasonable, or erroneous and misleading. This is where your background knowledge and a bit of healthy skepticism come into play. For respect of others' work, I have chosen not to provide articles that provide concrete examples of the types of miscalculations to look out for. Rather, I explain in some detail what to look for and what it may look like. I hope that you can still appreciate the skill of critiquing articles based on what is outlined in this chapter.

Why Is It Important to Critique Research Articles?

As I have already noted, most of our clinical decisions are based on information derived from empirical research. This empirical research should be based on decisive hypotheses, sound designs, and proper statistical models. A breach anywhere on this link undermines the credibility of the inferences. We can learn to offset these ruptures by developing skill at critiquing the research literature.

As clinical neuropsychologists, we are often making decisions about very serious matters—diagnoses, recommendations for treatment, prognoses, and interventions. It is important that we develop a greater appreciation for the work that goes behind these hefty decisions and remain well informed about how we generally arrive at these decisions that go beyond clinical lore and experience. However, case studies and clinical experience clearly have their value, but are also subject to biases that we might not be aware of.

It takes much more than reading through an article for improvement. Critiquing research articles is very different from reading, say, a science fiction book. The scientific method is not impervious to flaws, and it is a great skill to learn to be able to discern flaws and perhaps decide on your own what might have been more suitable. This skill will help you devise your own watertight research studies, detect potentially disabling mistakes with your own work, and most importantly, enhance the quality and credibility of your findings. But also, it will provide you with a different mindset, one that will become invaluable in your clinical work.

What Does It Take?

Reading through research articles takes a few fundamental skills. Primarily, one needs knowledge of research design and statistics. Don't worry. You need not know every little detail of factorial designs, or every single component of a regression analysis. On the other hand, you should have a general understanding of basic principles; the advantages and disadvantages of analysis of variance (ANOVA) over t-tests, the advantages and disadvantages of MANOVAs over ANOVAs, or even problems with certain data management strategies (e.g., dichotomizing continuous variables). However, many things to look out for may be methodological and not statistical.

How Will This Help Me?

The information provided in this chapter is intended to give you a little push. It is intended to give you an idea of the things you might pay more attention to while reading research articles. It is not uncommon to skip several subheadings of the Methods section because we simply do not understand the analyses involved, just do not care, or because the authors did a poor job at describing the analyses. Just as we are taught from day one, authors (and you, if you publish work) should have written the article so that others can glean enough information so that the readers would be able to replicate or refine that same study. In order to do so, the language must be clear and concrete, and the process of the study (as described throughout the Methods section) should be unambiguous. Authors should not assume that persons reading the article are familiar with all of the terminology or the statistics used. So, if you are using an unfamiliar or recondite method, provide a brief description so as not to bewilder your readers. The reasons for selecting such procedures, or even the very variables that were included, should be described. Any omissions can result in mind-numbing work for the readers as they must sift through the tables, figures, and results in an effort to determine what exactly the researchers examined, and worse, guess some of the particulars! Unfortunately, some authors engender frustration at the expense of highfalutin terminology and vague details.

You will be more inclined to find inconsistencies, problems with the design of the study or the statistics used for analyses. You might also realize that the conclusions reached are not substantiated by the authors' work, or that there were key issues the authors did not mention. You should also look at the figures and tables. Much like how you approach your own data during the preliminary stages prior to the main analysis. Does anything jump out at you? You should also question both what is committed and omitted. For example, if a good number of participants failed to return for follow up in a prospective study, did the authors demonstrate that they did or did not differ on certain variables—age, education, cognition, or the severity of an illness?

What I am saying is that it is important to go beyond the text. Thinking and reading critically is more effortful, but by engaging in such an active process of reading, you are more apt to remember and understand what you read at a deeper level. This is what will differentiate you from among the crowd.

Critiquing a research article should be done so systematically. Think of it as analogous to the inherent structure of a typical manuscript: Introduction, Methods, and Discussion sections. For each subsection, I have delineated problems that you might keep an eye out for. Keep in mind, these might range from the miniscule, such as grammatical errors, to the considerable, including gross conceptual misrepresentations, or distorting the interpretation of the analyses. Think of yourself as an editor. Use circumspection; be exacting and, do not be afraid to shake your head in disapproval with something you do not agree with despite an author's convincing conviction of the topic. This is not American Idol, you are not complimenting or insulting someone to his face. This is an art as much as it is a science. Language is important. Authors must say what they mean and mean what they say. Keep in mind that assuming such a frame of mind while reading research articles will come seamlessly with time. And, remember: read *beyond the text*—look at figures, tables, authors, affiliations, instruments, analyses, references, conflicts of interest, etc. And more importantly, try not to be so serious, and have a little fun.

Introduction

Much like the introduction to anything you have ever written, the introduction of a research article involves the "funnel" approach. Information about the topic proceeds from the broad to the specific. Authors are required to telescope vast amounts of information into a few paragraphs. For example, if you were to read an article on the neuropsychology of multiple sclerosis (MS), you will first encounter a statement about what MS is as well as the prevalence of cognitive deficits in MS. This introduces the reader to the topic, and then walks him or her along the author's intended path. The reader should be guiding you through gradually. A bad tour guide will have you hitting your head on branches, tripping over rocks, and eating sand. Perhaps he/she will also leave you alone and confused by the end of your trip! The goal of a writer is to enthrall readers—whether it is about the neuropsychology of MS or fishing (no offense). The reader should be able to understand how you arrive at each consecutive sentence, then at each paragraph, and ultimately, understand how the introduction culminates into the hypotheses of the study.

Other than the flow of the sentence, a carefully and deftly crafted introduction should choose words wisely. Confusing incidence and prevalence, correlation and causation, are examples of frequent blunders.

At times, authors will also use neuropsychological tests, but describe them as measuring a construct that we believe to be inaccurate—such as labeling Digit Span Forward as a measure of working memory (we generally consider this to be a measure of simple auditory attention).

At the end of the introduction, ask yourself whether the hypotheses make sense. Based on what the authors have taught you up until the end of the introduction section:

- Do the hypotheses of the study fit well?
- Are the hypotheses phrased appropriately?
- Do they use the term moderator when they mean mediator?
- Do they say predict when they mean classify?
- Do they say cause when they mean associate?

These are important distinctions. Refining neuropsychology as a science requires that we not only conceive novel hypotheses, but that we use the art of language accurately, and suitably apply the scientific method.

Method

Participants

The participants of a study affect several aspects of the study: the generalizability (external validity). Differences between groups of participants in a study are also important and can affect the interpretations.

Some basic questions you might ask yourself:

- From where do the participants come?
- Are the participants a heterogeneous group of patients, normal controls, or both, or a homogeneous subset of undergraduate psychology students?
- Are there demographic differences among groups in the sample?

- What is the make up of the group (s)?
- Are their differences in sex, ethnicity, education, or age?
- Is there something "odd" about the participants—is their mean education or IQ much higher than the general population?
- If this was a longitudinal study, how many participants did not return for follow up and how did they differ from the participants that returned?
- If there is a study on neuropsychological outcomes following surgery, do the authors use a proper control group (or a control group at all, such as a wait list control)? Do the authors (or you) recognize that persons chosen for neurosurgery are often qualitatively different from those who are not chosen to undergo surgery?
- If the patients are elders, does it make sense that men and women have similar levels of education? How common was it for women to complete college in the 30s, 40s, etc.? Therefore, if educational levels are roughly equivalent between sexes, does this suggest the women are qualitatively different from other women with fewer years of education, and does this limit the external validity of the results?

Anything that might represent a nuisance variable should be examined. A significant difference among groups on any variable that might explain a significant degree of variance in the dependent variables should be explored, and if present, managed. Naturally, researchers will compare differences among samples with statistical tests to determine whether the groups differ significantly on any one of these potential nuisance variables. If there are differences on one of these variables that could explain differences found between groups on the dependent variable, is it appropriate to include them as covariates? Is this a true experimental design (for which covariates are best suited for?). Does including education level when as a covariate when comparing persons with and without a psychiatric illness make sense? In other words, does the very fact that someone has a psychiatric illness limit their schooling?

Despite the fact that researchers will inform you of whether nuisance variables differ between the groups, it is always wise to examine the descriptive statistics for all variables that are presented in the tables. Just because there are no significant differences among variables, you can still glean valuable information from the data. You can look at the means and standard deviations of the variables. Is one of the standard deviations much greater than all others? Is there a trend in the data, despite the fact that there are no significant findings? Do the numbers make sense, that is, do patients with Alzheimer disease score more poorly on a memory test than patients with mild cognitive impairment and cognitively normal controls? Do the authors consider p-values of 0.05 significant even after multiple tests, resulting in an increased probability of a type I error? Do the authors appreciate the difference between an association and a manipulation/causation? In fact, even when groups are randomly selected, it might be that if patient groups are not randomly assigned, those who are considered in need of more aggressive treatment will be placed in a treatment group that is in and of itself "more aggressive."

Another thing to consider is whether the patient groups are a good representation of the population from which they come. For example, it would be unlikely for persons with a chronic mental illness to have (as a group) an overall IQ in the average range. This might mean that these patients are higher functioning than most persons with illness, and therefore, it would be difficult to extrapolate or generalize the findings to patients with the same illness who did not participate in the study.

Materials/Apparatus

Of course, the authors will be examining one or more hypothetical constructs; memory, attention, depression, etc. And, we use scales, inventories, and tests to operationally define these hypothetical constructs. We use performance (scores) from these measures to infer the integrity of cognition or the severity of an affective illness. If we are to infer the integrity of a cognitive domain, and perhaps, the associated pathophysiology or neuroanatomical correlates, it is important that tests are used accordingly.

We often describe what tests do, rather than what they actually measure. For example, for the Trail Making Test, we might say that it is a measure of visual attention, visual tracking, or psychomotor processing speed. The truth is, this test includes all three (and probably more) of these abilities. However, it is often presumptuous to state what a test measures, because tests measure different things in different patients and in different populations. In other words, someone who has oculomotor impairments, such as patients with progressive supranuclear palsy, might do poorly on the Trail Making Test because of poor visual scanning. Patients who have Parkinson's disease might do poorly because of their profound bradykinesia (slowed movements).

Think about the data from the tests as well. Is the test used one that is not commonly normally distributed, yet the authors are using parametric tests. Should they have used nonparametric tests or transformed the data?

Procedure

The procedure has to do with the process of what the patients and controls went through during the study. So, if this was a repeated measures design, see whether the tests were counterbalanced. Were patients remunerated for their participation? If so, did they receive similar amounts of money for each session (if it was a longitudinal design)?

Figures

Check whether the figures are scaled appropriately. Do the axes reflect gradations in a variable so as to unintentionally (or perhaps intentionally) magnify the effects?

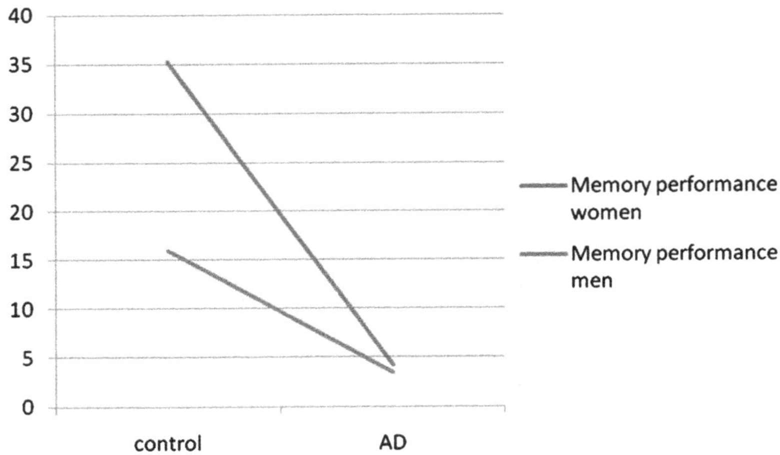

Fig. 10.1 Factorial ANOVA

Did the authors use a figure that is misleading or mispresentative of the findings, or of the value of the findings? For example, look at Fig. 10.1. The variables indicate this is a between-subjects design: men in the control and AD group, and women in the control and AD group. However, the graph suggests that scores are declining, whereas it merely indicates that both men and women who have AD perform more poorly on tests of memory, and that control women perform better than control men!!

Discussion Section

The discussion section is probably the most challenging portion of a manuscript to write. It is here that authors must synthesize the results of their own study, interpret the statistical analyses, and dovetail all of this information with the background history. At times, the findings of your study will parallel the work of many others. However, it is not uncommon that your findings will contradict those of other studies, or perhaps, not make intuitive sense. As you can see, this section requires a great deal of creativity and even additional hypothesis testing.

First, see if the authors summed up the gist of the article that is an accurate reflection of what you were able to glean from reading else. Do they discuss the most salient limitations of the study that you were able to discern while reading through the paper?

Title

So, you have perused and parsed the entire article, now it is time to take it to the third level; presumptuousness. The last question to ask yourself is: "does the title accurately reflect the content, findings, and purpose of the article?" If yes, great, but, another great exercise is to think of an alternative title that is perhaps more precise. Is the current title of the article misleading? Does it place emphasis on something that is given short shrift in the manuscript?

Think of the abstract as seeing the preview to a movie. Imagine that after a 2-min trailer of gun slinging, fast cars, and drugs, 99% of the actual movie involved romantic dinners.

Think of the title of a movie similar to that of a manuscript's title. So, for the previous example, it might be misleading if the movie were called, "smash it up," when in fact, it might have been more accurate to have entitled the movie, "love and kisses."

As another example, is the title, "The effect of cognition on activities of daily living," accurate when the study is merely one of association and not causation? Therefore, you might suggest (to yourself, that is) a new title: "Cognitive function is associated with activities of daily living." It may not be eloquent, but it is definitely more accurate.

A rule of thumb to capture an accurate title for your manuscript is to try to use the independent and dependent variables used within the study. For example, if the authors examined the effect of alcohol (the independent variable) on gait (the dependent variable), the title of the manuscript might be, "Impairments in gait as a function of alcohol intake." Often, the significant findings in the article (and at times the results which are inconsequential) are extrapolated and underscored in the title. So, among several analyses, only those that are relevant to the findings are reflected in the title.

A Change in Roles

As you can see, it is easy to find flaws in research, that is because no study is without them. However, the talent lies in one's ability to generate alternative ideas of how the authors might have studied differently the phenomenon of interest. This is in part an academic exercise, but requires a more refined understanding of experimental design.

There are three main areas that might help to refine your ability to refine a study: the design, analysis, and the conclusions/inferences of the findings.

The Design

This part forms the crux of true experimental work. It requires substantial ingenuity and forethought. The design includes the participants in the study (the control and experimental groups), how the tests were administered (and in what order), as well as the type and number of instruments and materials used.

Most think of an ideal control group as free of disease or infirmary. However, the purpose of a control group is to "control" for things *other than* the variable (e.g., disease) of primary interest. For example, if the purpose of a study was to compare patients on an inpatient unit who recently suffered a stroke, perhaps inpatients who have not suffered strokes but share several common features—inpatient stay, a large number of medicines, pain, etc. would be ideal.

Tests serve as proxies for the phenomena under study. If they do not have established reliability and validity—or are not in line with what the authors were purportedly studying—then selecting more appropriate measures (e.g., paired-associated learning instead of list learning), or additional measures (e.g., brain imaging, psychological variables such as personality and mood disorders).

The Analysis

This part has to do with the statistical analysis (or analyses) chosen to examine the hypothesis (or hypotheses). For example, did the authors dichotomize a variable when in fact the analysis might have revealed more sensitive and valuable information had the variables be left alone? So, perhaps persons on a questionnaire of depression were considered either depressed or not depressed by using a median split to define the groups. On the other hand, it is often more useful to use the values as a continuous variable and examine them accordingly. Of course, there are instances where it makes sense to dichotomize variables (e.g., a restricted range of scores), but this is something you should be able to determine by examining the descriptive statistics provided by the authors.

Inferences

There are generally several interpretations proffered after the results of the analysis. Some might be far stretched (and far fetched) in an effort for the authors to "make excuses" for why they might have yielded inconsistent, unpredicted, and unlikely results. It is helpful to write down your own inferences on a piece of paper before reading through the authors'. You can then compare and contrast what you have learned from what the authors are reporting. Sometimes it is a matter of what the authors want to emphasize and de-emphasize. For example, for patients who underwent a particular surgical procedure, 15% of whom developed postoperative cognitive decline. If the authors ascribed to the tenets of evidence-based practice, and had a patient who was very similar to the research participants, the clinician may tell the person that he or she has a 15% chance of postoperative cognitive decline (as extrapolated from the study), or that 85% of persons who undergo this surgery demonstrate no objective evidence of cognitive decline following surgery.

Summary

My hope is that you have read through this chapter and gained a better appreciation for the effort involved in reading through even one scientific article. The reader's job is to question the precision of each and every word, each and every table, and each and every figure. As much as these are academic exercises, the aim is to be more proficient in both study and ultimate practice of clinical neuropsychology.

I also hope that you now read everything with a grain of salt; don't assume that what other authors are discussing is entirely accurate. Double-check some of the information with other sources including mine.

Bibliography

Anastasi, A. (1950). The concept of validity in the interpretation of test scores. *Educational and Psychological Measurement, 10*, 67–78.

Andreasen, N. C. (1983). *Scale for the assessment of negative symptoms*. Iowa City: University of Iowa Press.

Andreasen, N. C. (1984). *Scale for the assessment of positive symptoms*. Iowa City: University of Iowa Press.

Beck, A. T., Ward, C. H., Mendelson, M., Mock, J., & Erbaugh, J. (1961). An inventory for measuring depression. *Archives of General Psychiatric, 4*, 51–571.

Benedict, R. H. B., Cookfair, D., Gavett, R., Gunther, M., Munschauer, F., Garg, N., et al. (2006). Validity of the minimal assessment of cognition function in multiple sclerosis (MACFIMS). *Journal of the International Neuropsychological Society, 12*. 549–558.

Box, G. E. P. (1949). A general distribution theory for a class of likelihood criteria. *Biometrika, 36*, 317–346.

Brandt, J., & Benedict, R. H. B. (2001). *Hopkins verbal learning test-revised*. Lutz, FL: Psychological Assessment Resources.

Brooks, B. L., Strauss, E., Sherman, E. M. S., Iverson, G. L., & Slick, D. J. (2009). Developments in neuropsychological assessment: Refining psychometric and clinical interpretive methods. Canadian Psychology, 50(3), 196–209.

Bryant, F. B. (2000). Assessing the validity of measurement. In L. G., Grimm & P. R. Yarnold (Eds.), *Reading and understanding more multivariate statistics* (pp. 99–146). Washington, DC: American Psychological Association.

Budd, M. A., Kortte, K. B., Cloutman, L., Newhart, M., Gottesman, R. F., Davis, C., Heidler-Gary, J., Seay, M. W., Hillis, A. E. (2010). The nature of naming errors in primary progressive aphasia versus acute post-stroke aphasia. Neuropsychology, 24(5), 581–589.

Busch, R. M., Chelune, G. J., & Suchy, Y. (2006). Using norms in neuropsychological assessment of the elderly. In D. K. Attix & K. A. Welsh-Bohmer (Eds.), *Geriatric neuropsychology*. New York: The Guilford Press.

Busch, R. M., Frazier, T. W., Haggerty, K. A., & Kubu, C. S. (2005). Utility of the Boston naming test in predicting ultimate side of surgery in patients with medically intractable temporal lobe epilepsy. *Epilepsia, 46*, 1773–1779.

Butcher, J. N., Graham, J. R., Ben-Porath, Y. S., Tellegen, A., Dahlstrom, W. G., & Kaemmer, B. (2001). *MMPI-2: Manual for administration and scoring* (Rev.th ed.). Minneapolis: University of Minnesota Press.

D.A. Maroof, *Statistical Methods in Neuropsychology: Common Procedures Made Comprehensible*, DOI 10.1007/978-1-4614-3417-7,

Campbell, D. T., & Fiske, D. W. (1959). Convergent and discriminant validation by the multitrait-multimethod matrix. *Psychological Bulletin, 56*, 81–105.

Catell, R. B. (1966). The scree test for the number of factors. *Multivariate Behavioral Research, 1*, 245–276.

Chaytor, N., & Schmitter-Edgecombe, M. (2003). The ecological validity of neuropsychological tests: A review of the literature on everyday cognitive skills. *Neuropsychology Review, 13*, 181–197.

Cohen, J. (1992). A power primer. *Psychological bulletin, 112*, 155–159.

Costello, A. B., & Osborne, J. W. (2005). Best practices in exploratory factor analysis: Four recommendations for getting the most from your analysis. *Practical Assessment, Research Evaluation, 10*, 1–9.

Cronbach, L. J. (1951). Coefficient alpha and the internal structure of tests. *Psychometrika, 16*, 297–334.

Cullum, C. M., Weiner, M. F., & Saine, K. C. (2009). *Texas functional living scale examiner's manual*. San Antonio, TX: Pearson.

DeVellis, R. F. (2003). *Scale development: Theory and applications* (2nd ed., Vol. 26). *Applied social research methods series*. Newbury Park, CA: Sage.

Fabrigar, L. R., Wegener, D. T., MacCallum, R. C., & Strahan, E. J. (1999). Evaluating the use of exploratory factor analysis in psychological research. *Psychological Methods, 4*, 272–299.

Folstein, M. F., Folstein, S. E., & McHugh, P. R. (1975). Mini-mental state: Practical method for grading the cognitive state of patients for the clinician. *Journal of Psychiatric Research, 12*, 189–198.

Ford, J. K., MacCallum, R. C., & Tait, M. (1986). The application of exploratory factor analysis in applied psychology: A critical review and analysis. *Personnel Psychology, 39*, 291–314.

Franzen, M. D., & Wilhelm, K. L. (1996). Conceptual foundations of ecological validity in neuropsychology. In R. J. Sbordone & C. J. Long (Eds.), *Ecological validity of neuropsychological testing* (pp. 91–112). Lucie Press, Delray Beach, FL: GR press/St.

Geoergy D. and Mallery P. 2007. SPSS for Windows step by step: A simple guide and reference. 6th edition, Pearson Educations, Delhi, India.

Green, S. B. & Salkind, N. J. (2005). Using SPSS for windows and Macintosh: Analyzing and understanding data (4th ed.). Pearson Prentice Hall: New Jersey

Guttman, L. (1954). Some necessary conditions for common-factor analysis. *Psychometrika, 19*, 149–161.

Harlow, L. L. (2005). *The essence of multivariate thinking: Basic themes and methods*. Mahwah, NJ: Lawrence Erlbaum Associates.

Harris, R. J. (2001). *A primer of multivariate statistics* (3rd ed.). Mahwah, New Jersey: Lawrence Erlbaum Associates.

Hayton, J. C., Allen, D. G., & Scarpello, V. (2004). Factor retention decisions in exploratory factor analysis: A tutorial on parallel analysis. *Organizational Research Methods, 7*, 191–205.

Holm, S. (1979). A simple sequentially rejective multiple test procedure. *Scandinavian Journal of Statistics, 6*, 65–70.

Holtzer, R., Goldin, Y., Zimmerman, M., Katz, M., Buschke, H., & Lipton, R. B. (2008). Robust norms for selected neuropsychological tests in older adults. *Archives of Clinical Neuropsychology, 23*, 531–541.

Horn, J. L. (1965). A rationale and test for the number of factors in factor analysis. *Psychometrica, 30*, 179–185.

Huberty, C. J., & Morris, J. D. (1989). Multivariate analysis versus multiple univariate analyses. *Psychological Bulletin, 105*, 302–308.

Kaiser, H. F. (1960). The application of electronic computers to factor analysis. *Educational and Psychological Measurement, 20*, 141–151.

Kaplan, E., Goodglass, H., & Weintrab, S. (1983). *The Boston naming test*. Philadelphia: Lea & Febiger.

Larsen, R., & Warne, R. T. (2010). Estimating confidence intervals for eigenvalues in exploratory factor analysis. *Behavior Research Methods, 42*, 871–876.

Licht, M. H. (2001). Multiple regressino and correlation. In Reading and understanding multivariate statistics (2001). Grimm, L.G. & Yarnold, P.R. American Psychological Association.

Morey, L. C. (1991). *The personality assessment Inventory professional manual*. Odessa, FL: Psychological Assessment Resources.

Nunnally, J. C., & Bernstein, I. H. (1994). *Psychometric theory* (3rd ed.). New York: McGraw-Hill.

Parmenter et al. (2010). The utility of regression-based norms in interpreting the minimal assessment of cognitive function in multiple sclerosis (MACFIMS). Journal of the International Neuropsychological Society, 16, 6–16.

Pauker, J. D. (1988). Constructing overlapping cell tables to maximize the clinical usefulness of normative test data: Rationale and an example from neuropsychology. *Journal of Clinical Psychology, 44*, 930–933.

Porter, A. C., & Raudenbush, S. W. (1987). Analysis of covariance: Its model and use in psychological research. *Journal of Counseling Psychology, 34*, 383–392.

Randolph, C. (1998). *Repeatable battery for the assessment of neuropsychological status: Manual*. San Antonio, TX: The Psychological Corporation.

Schoenberg, M. R., Duff, K., Scott, J. G., Patton, D., & Adams, R. L. (2006). Prediction errors of the Oklahoma premorbid intelligence estimate–3 (OPIE-3) stratified by 13 age groups. *Archives of Clinical Neuropsychology, 21*, 469–475.

Sliwinski, M., Lipton, R. B., Buschke, H., & Stewart, W. (1996). The effects of preclinical dementia on estimates of normal cognitive functioning in aging. *Journal of Gerontology Series B: Psychological Sciences and Social Science, 51*, P217–P225.

Stevens, J. P. (2002). *Applied multivariate statistics for the social sciences* (4th ed.). Mahwah, NJ: Lawrence Erlbaum Associates, Publishers.

Strauss, E., Sherman, E., Spreen, O. (2006). A compendium of neuropsychological tests: Administration, norms, and commentary. 3rd edition. NY Oxford University Press.

Tabachnick, B. G., & Fidell, L. S. (2001). *Using multivariate statistics* (4th ed.). Needham Heights, MA: Allyn and Bacon.

Testa, S. M., Winicki, J. M., Pearlson, G. D., Gordon, B., & Schretlen, D. J. (2009). Accounting for estimated IQ in neuropsychological test performance with regression-based techniques. *Journal of the International Neuropsychological Society, 15*, 1012–1022.

The Psychological Corporation. (2001). *Manual for the wechsler test of adult reading (WTAR)*. San Antonio: The Psychological Corporation.

Velicer, W. F., & Jackson, D. N. (1990). Component analysis versus common factor-analysis–Some further observations. *Multivariate Behavioral Research, 25*, 97–114.

Wright, R. E. (1995). Logistic regression. In L. G. Grimm & P. R. Yarnold (Eds.), *Reading and Understanding More Multivariate Statistics* (pp. 217–244). Washington, DC: American Psychological Association.

Zimet, G. D., Dahlem, N. W., Zimet, S. G., & Farley, G. K. (1988). The multidimensional scale of perceived social support. *Journal of Personality Assessment, 52*, 30–41.

Index

D.A. Maroof, *Statistical Methods in Neuropsychology: Common Procedures Made Comprehensible*, DOI 10.1007/978-1-4614-3417-7,

www.ingramcontent.com/pod-product-compliance
Lightning Source LLC
Chambersburg PA
CBHW071801310326
42187CB00003B/148
9781461434160